HATHA YOGA

Contact: oneofakindbooks@bhagwan.se

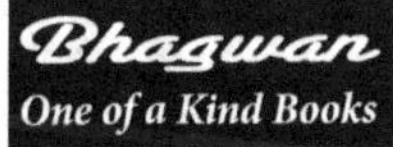

Bhagwan
One of a Kind Books

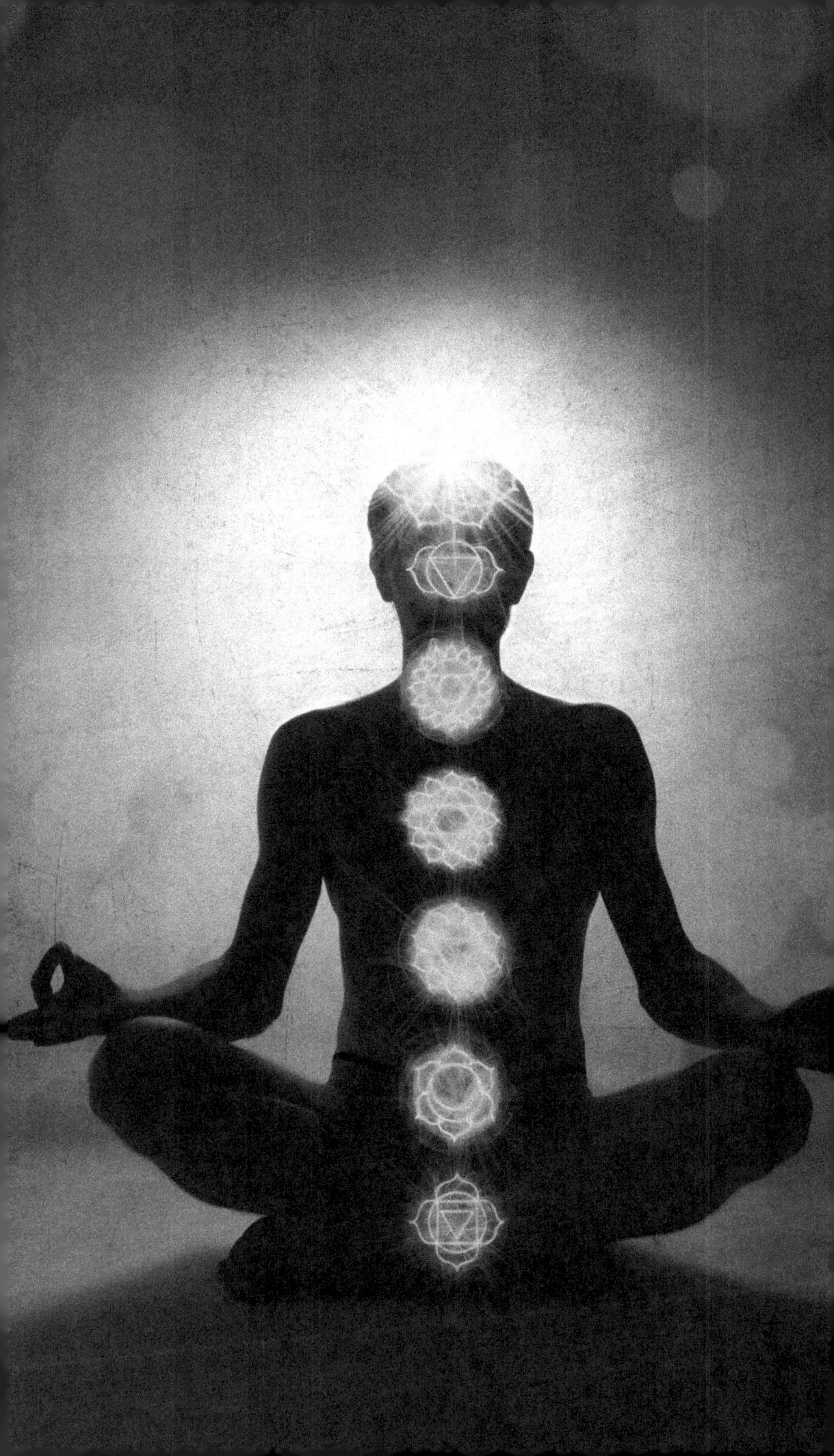

HATHA YOGA

ISBN 9789180206259

❋❋❋

The

HATHA YOGA PRADIPIKA

Introduced by Shreyananda Natha

Contact: oneofakindbooks@bhagwan.se

Publisher: **BHAGWAN 2021**

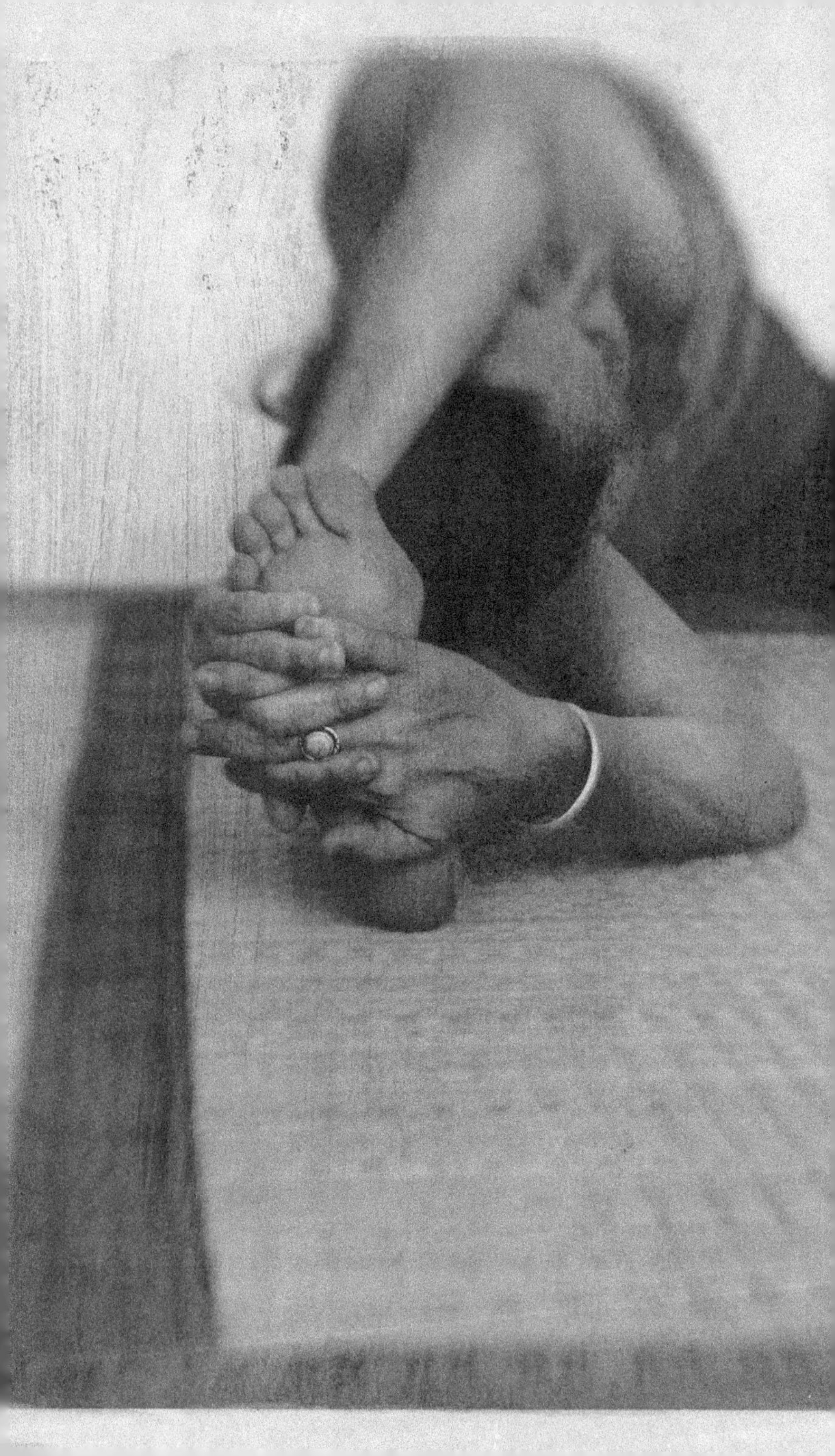

"As one opens the door with a key, so the yogi should
open the gate to liberation with the kundalini.

The great goddess sleeps, closing with her mouth,
the opening through which one can ascend to the
Brahmarandhra…
to that place where there is neither pain nor suffering.

The kundalini sleeps above the kanda…
she gives liberation to the yogi and bondage to the fool.

He who knows kundalini, knows yoga.

The kundalini, it is said, is coiled like a serpent.
He who can induce her to move is liberated."

Hatha Yoga Pradipika v. 105-111.

Index

Introduction by Shreyananda Natha. *Page 8*

Chapter 1: ASANAS. *Page 19*

Chapter 2: PRANAYAMAS. *Page 45*

Chapter 3: MUDRAS. *Page 79*

Chapter 4: SAMADHI. *Page 123*

Introduction

Hatha Yoga Pradipika.

Is the No.1 most read book about yoga besides Patanjalis Yogasutras. The Hatha Yoga Pradipika, along with the Gheranda-Samhita (1650), is one of the most detailed manuals describing the techniques of Hatha Yoga. The book is the hatha yoga text that has historically been studied within yoga teacher training programmes, alongside texts on classical yoga such as Patanjali's Yoga Sutras.

The HYP is a medieval yoga text, dating from about the 15th or 16th century, and is as much about Tantra as about Yoga. It was compiled by Swātmārama. It´s name means "special (pra) light (dipika) on forceful (hatha) yoga". It is much later in date than the Yoga Sutras, and provides details of Hatha Yoga techniques which the Yoga Sutras don't touch on. But there are also occasional sutras which touch on familiar concerns (for example, compare HYP 4.23 with YS 1.2). It is just about yoga practice, as contrasted with the Bhagavad Gītā, which is about how to live in the everyday world.

The word "hatha" requires a little comment. The concept

is that we live in an energy field; energy is behind all action. The energy field that we live in normally extends 4 fingers-breadth beyond the body, and it is possible also in a healthy person to achieve a situation in which the energy is concentrated inside the body. In an unhealthy person the energy dissipates further. There are blockages in an unhealthy person that makes it impossible to concentrate one's energy properly, and techniques such as nadi śodhana are used to open the channels and improve the flow of energy.

There is in fact a whole complex of energy channels or nādī within the body, of which there are 11 primary nadi, coming from a central hub (kanda) located in the lower abdomen, and branching out into many others (traditionally, 72,000).

There are 10 nadi associated with perception and action:

eyes (sight)

tongue (speech)

ears (hearing)

fingers & thumbs (grasping)

tongue (taste)

big toes (locomotion)

skin (feeling)

bladder & anus (excretion)

nostrils (smell)

sex organs (generation)

If the quality of the nadi is poor, the quality of perception and action is also poor.

There is one more nadi, the susumna, which instead of flowing out, flows in, linking us to the inner world. It runs from the kanda to the base of the spine then to the top of the head. There are two processes in energy, ha and tha, which flow through the pingala and ida channels (or nādī) respectively, and then unite to flow into susumna. Usually it is not possible for energy to flow into susumna because of a blockage at the base of the spine. The practice of Hatha Yoga tries to create a state of breakthrough allowing energy to flow into susumna, bringing with it a stable state of mind. The Hatha Yoga Pradipika teaches techniques that allow this state to be achieved.

The difference between the Hatha Yoga of the Hatha Yoga Pradipika and the Raja Yoga of the Yoga Sutras is that Hatha Yoga uses prana as a primary working tool, whereas Raja Yoga uses the mind as its primary working tool. These days very few people are able to practice Hatha Yoga sufficiently strongly for it to work properly.

The key ideas in the text are:

Chapter 1 – āsana: used to stimulate energy (prana);
Chapter 2 – prānāyāma: used to contain/condense energy;
Chapter 3 – mudrā: used to direct energy;
Chapter 4 – dhyāna: used to integrate and merge energy.

Chapter Summaries:

CHAPTER 1: Asanas.
1-11 Introduction.
Hatha yoga "shines forth as a stairway to raja yoga" (1); is "the greatest secret of the yogis who wish to attain perfection".
12-16 Conditions for practice.
The "hermitage" described (12-14); obstacles and supports (15-16). The ten yama and ten niyama in sutras 16ii and 16iii are apparently later additions to the text; hatha yoga does not in fact place much emphasis on them.

17-56 Āsana.

The role of āsana is to develop steadiness of body and mind, flexibility of the limbs; sequence for practice is āsana → prāṇāyāma → mudrā → meditation (56).

57-63 Diet and Restrictions.

Mitāhāra – appropriate food (57, 62-63); food to avoid (58-59); other things to avoid (60-61).

64-67 Conclusion.

Importance of practical application emphasised (64-66); hatha yoga leads to Raja Yoga (67).

CHAPTER 2: Prāṇāyāmas.

1-3 Breath and mind.

First make the body steady, then bring steadiness to prāna (1); when prāna moves, citta moves (2).

4-5 Nāḍī and malā.

Nadīs must be purified so that prāna can flow.

6-20 Practice guidelines.

Practice daily (6); nadi śodhana (7-12); milk and ghee important foods (14); negative effects of inappropriate practice (15-17); indications of purification (18-20).

21-36 The Śat Karma (cleansing techniques).

These should be practised only by persons with kapha imbalance (21).

37-74 Prāṇāyāma.

Some teachers say prāṇāyāma alone is enough to cleanse the system (37); prāṇāyāma purifies the nādīs and chakras, and opens the door to suśumna (41); manon-mani – mind devoid of thought (42); eight types of kum-bhaka (43-70); three processes of prāṇāyāma (71-74); two processes of kumbhaka (72-74).

75-77 Kundalini and Raja Yoga.

By practising kumbhaka, kundalini is aroused and suśumna is freed of obstacles (75); both hatha and raja yoga are essential for perfection (samādhi) (76).

78 Eight signs of perfection.

lean body, bright face, strong voice, clear eyes, no disease, control of semen, active digestive fire, purification of nā-dis.

CHAPTER 3: Mudrās.

1-2 Kundalini.

Kundalini the support of all yoga practices.

3-5 Susumnā.

When kundalini awakens, susumnā becomes pathway of prāna (3); the "goddess sleeping at Brahma's door" can be aroused by performing mudrā.

6-103 Ten mudrās described.

10-18 maha mudra.

19-25 maha bandha.

26-29 maha vedha.

30-31 when to perform these three.

32-54 khechari mudra.

55-60 uddiyana bandha.

61-69 mula bandha.

70-73 jalandhara bandha.

74-77 comments on the three bandhas.

78-82 viparita karani.

83-91 vajroli mudra.

92-95 sahajoli mudra.

96-103 maroli mudra.

104-124 Kundalini.

Kundalini is coiled like a snake(108), 3½ times, at base of susumnā; you have to awaken the snake (111) [like getting rid of a snake in a tree by either hitting the tree with a stick or lighting a fire under it]; this moves kundalini so that it is drawn up into susumnā a little way (117), thus allowing prāna to enter susumnā (118). Best way to do this is to practise bhastrika with kumbhaka (122); other than arousing kundalini, the other way to purify the nadis including susumnā is regular practice of āsana, prānāyāma, mudrā and concentration (124).

125-127 Importance of mental attitude.

Prānāyāma should be practised with a focused mind.

128-130 Conclusion.

CHAPTER 4: Samādhi.

1-9 Samādhi.

Mind and ātman come together in samādhi.

10-29 Prāna.

When prāna flows in susumnā, the mind is blank (12);

as well as prāna, air and fire enter suśumnā (19); when mind is still, prāna is suspended, when prāna is suspended, mind is still (23); if they are controlled, moksa (liberation) is attained (25); this brings steadiness to the body (28).

30-34 Laya (dissolution)

Definition of laya (31).

35-37 Śambhavi mudra (eyebrow centre gazing).

38-47 Khecari.

48 Tūrya.

This "fourth state" is one in which the mind is quiescent.

49-53 Yoga Nidrā.

This is the state in which the conscious mind subsides but awareness remains. It's like a pot filled with space (50).

54-63 Samādhi.

64-102 Nāda.

The sound created by the union of Śiva and Śakti.

Four stages of yoga practice (69-77).

Raja yoga (78-79).

Modern research.

The Hatha Yoga Pradipika is the hatha yoga text that has historically been studied within yoga teacher training programmes, alongside texts on classical yoga such as Patanjali's Yoga Sutras. In the twenty-first century, research on the history of yoga has led to a more developed understanding of hatha yoga's origins.

James Mallinson has studied the origins of hatha yoga in classic yoga texts such as the Khecarīvidyā. He has identified eight works of early hatha yoga that may have contributed to its official formation in the Hatha Yoga Pradipika. This has stimulated further research into understanding the formation of hatha yoga.

Jason Birch has investigated the role of the Hatha Yoga Pradīpikā in popularizing an interpretation of the Sanskrit word hatha. The text drew from classic texts on different systems of yoga, and Svātmārāma grouped what he had found under the generic term "hatha yoga". Examining Buddhist tantric commentaries and earlier medieval yoga texts, Birch found that the adverbial uses of the word suggested that it meant "force", rather than "the metaphysical explanation proposed in the 14th century Yogabīja of uniting the sun (ha) and moon (tha.

The Hatha Yoga Pradipika is also an ocean of secret/hidden knowledge.

Seeker. Listen to this vers:

*"As one opens the door with a key, so the yogi should
open the gate to liberation with the kundalini.*

*The great goddess sleeps, closing with her mouth,
the opening through which one can ascend to the Brah-
marandhra...
to that place where there is neither pain nor suffering.*

*The kundalini sleeps above the kanda...
she gives liberation to the yogi and bondage to the fool.*

He who knows kundalini, knows yoga.

*The kundalini, it is said, is coiled like a serpent.
He who can induce her to move is liberated."*

Hatha Yoga Pradipika v. 105-111.

Om Sri Durgayai Namah

*Remebering we are one. Be always united with the force
of the universe. She will take care about you but not for
free. Remember this.*

Yogi Shreyananda Natha

Chapter 1

ASANAS

Prathamopadeśah

1.) śrī-ādi-nāthāya namo|astu tasmai yeno-
padiṣhṭā haṭha-yogha-vidyā | vibhrājate
pronnata-rāja-yogham āroḍhumichchorad-
hirohiṇīva

*Salutations to Shiva, who taught the science of Hatha
Yoga.*
It is the aspirant's stairway to the heights of Raja Yoga.

2.) praṇamya śrī-ghuruṃ nāthaṃ svātmārā-
meṇa yoghinā | kevalaṃ rāja-yoghāya
haṭha-vidyopadiśyate

*Yogi Svatmarama, after saluting the Lord and guru,
explains the science of Hatha for one reason – Raja
Yoga.*

3.) bhrāntyā bahumata-dhvānte rāja-yogha-
majānatām | haṭha-pradīpikāṃ dhatte svāt-
mārāmaḥ kṛpākaraḥ

*For those ignorant of Raja Yoga, wandering in the dark-
ness of too many opinions, compassionate Svatmarama
gives the light of Hatha.*

**4.) haṭha-vidyāṃ hi matsyendra-ghorakṣhā-
dyā vijānate | svātmārāmo|athavā yoghī
jānīte tat-prasādataḥ**

*Matsyendra, Goraksha, and others know well the science
of Hatha. By their grace, Yogi Svatmarama also knows
it.*

*The following Siddhas (masters) are said to have existed
in former times. Guru–shishya means "succession from
Guru to disciple". Paramparā literally means an unin-
terrupted row or series, order, succession, continuation,
mediation, tradition.*

**5.) śrī-ādinātha-matsyendra-śāvarānan-
da-bhairavāḥ | chaurangghī-mīna-gho-
rakṣha-virūpākṣha-bileśayāḥ**

*Sri Âdinâtha (Śiva), Matsyendra, Nâtha, Sâbar, Anand,
Bhairava, Chaurangi, Mîna nâtha, Goraksanâtha,
Virupâksa, Bileśaya.*

**6.) manthāno bhairavo yoghī siddhirbudd-
haścha kanthaḍiḥ | koraṃṭakaḥ surānandaḥ
siddhapādaścha charpaṭiḥ**

*Manthâna, Bhairava, Siddhi Buddha, Kanthadi, Karan-
taka, Surânanda, Siddhipâda, Charapati.*

7.) kānerī pūjyapādaścha nitya-nātho nirañjanaḥ | kapālī bindunāthaścha kākachaṇḍīśvarāhvayaḥ

Kânerî, Pûjyapâda, Nityanâtha, Nirañjana, Kapâli, Vindunâtha, Kâka Chandîśwara.

8.) allāmaḥ prabhudevaścha ghoḍā cholī cha ṭiṃṭiṇiḥ | bhānukī nāradevaścha khaṇḍaḥ kāpālikastathā

Allâma, Prabhudeva, Ghodâ, Cholî, Tintini, Bhânukî Nârdeva, Khanda Kâpâlika, etc.

9.) ityādayo mahāsiddhā haṭha-yogha-prabhā-vataḥ | khaṇḍayitvā kāla-daṇḍaṃ brahmāṇḍe vicharanti te

These Mahâsiddhas (great masters), having conquered death through the power of Hatha Yoga, roam the universe.

10.) aśeṣha-tāpa-taptānāṃ samāśraya-maṭho haṭhaḥ | aśeṣha-yogha-yuktānāmādhāra-ka-maṭho haṭhaḥ

Hatha is the sanctuary for those suffering every type of pain.

*It is the foundation for those practicing every type of
Yoga.*

11.) haṭha-vidyā paraṃ ghopyā yoghinā siddhimichchhatā | bhavedvīryavatī ghuptā nirvīryā tu prakāśitā

*A Yogî desirous of success should keep the knowledge of
Hatha Yoga secret; for it becomes potent by concealing,
and impotent by exposing.*

12.) surājye dhārmike deśe subhikṣhe ni-rupadrave | dhanuḥ pramāṇa-paryantaṃ śilāghni-jala-varjite | ekānte maṭhikā-madhye sthātavyaṃ haṭha-yoghinā

*The Yogî should practise Hatha Yoga in a small room,
situated in a solitary place, being 4 cubits square, and
free from stones, fire, water, disturbances of all kinds,
and in a country where justice is properly administered,
where good people live, and food can be obtained easily
and plentifully.*

13.) alpa-dvāramarandhra-gharta-vivaraṃ nātyuchchha-nīchāyataṃ samyagh-gho-maya-sāndra-liptamamalaṃ niḥśesa-jantūjjhi-tam | bāhye maṇḍapa-vedi-kūpa-ruchiraṃ

**prākāra-saṃveṣhṭitaṃ proktaṃ yog-
ha-maṭhasya lakṣhaṇamidaṃ siddhair-
haṭhābhyāsibhiḥ**

*The room should have a small door, be free from holes,
hollows, neither too high nor too low, well plastered
with cow-dung and free from dirt, filth and insects.
On its outside there should be bowers, raised platform
(chabootrâ), a well, and a compound. These characte-
ristics of a room for Hatha Yogîs have been described by
adepts in the practice of Hatha.*

**14.) aevaṃ vidhe maṭhe sthitvā sar-
va-chintā-vivarjitaḥ | ghurūpadiṣhṭa-mārg-
heṇa yoghameva samabhyaset**

*Having seated in such a room and free from all anxie-
ties, he should practise Yoga, as instructed by his Guru.*

**15.) atyāhāraḥ prayāsaścha prajalpo niy-
amāghrahaḥ | jana-sangghaścha laulyaṃ
cha ṣhaḍbhiryogho vinaśyati**

*Yoga perishes by these six: overeating, overexertion,
talking too much, performing needless austerities, soci-
al-izing, and restlessness.*

16.) utsāhātsāhasāddhairyāttattva-jñānāścha niśchayāt | jana-sanggha-parityāg- hātṣhaḍbhiryoghaḥ prasiddhyati

Yoga succeeds by these six: enthusiasm, openness, coura- ge, knowledge of the truth, determination, and solitude.

17.) atha yama-niyamāḥ ahiṃsā satyamastey- am brahmacharyaṃ kṣhamā dhṛtiḥ | dayārja- vaṃ mitāhāraḥ śauchaṃ chaiva yamā daśa

The ten rules of conduct are: ahimsâ (non-injuring), truth, non-stealing, continence, forgiveness, endurance, compassion, meekness, sparing diet and cleanliness.

18.) tapaḥ santoṣha āstikyaṃ dānamīśva- ra-pūjanam | siddhānta-vākya-śravaṇaṃ hrīmatī cha tapo hutam | niyamā daśa samproktā yogha-śāstra-viśāradaiḥ

The ten niyamas mentioned by those proficient in the knowledge of yoga are: Tapa, patience, belief in God, charity, adoration of God, hearing discourses on the principles of religion, shame, intellect, Tapa and Yajña.

19.) atha āsanam haṭhasya prathamānggghat- vādāsanaṃ pūrvamuchyate | kuryāttadāsa- naṃ sthairyamāroghyaṃ chānggha-lāghavam

Being the first accessory of Hatha Yoga, âsana is described first. It should be practised for gaining steady posture, health and lightness of body.

20.) vaśiṣhṭhādyaiścha munibhirmatsyendrā-dyaiścha yoghibhiḥ ǀ angghīkṛtānyāsanāni kathyante kānichinmayā

I am going to describe certain âsanas which have been adopted by Munîs like Vasistha and Yogîs like Matsyendra.

21.) jānūrvorantare samyakkṛtvā pāda-tale ubhe ǀ r̥ju-kāyaḥ samāsīnaḥ svastikaṃ tat-prachakṣhate

Swastika-âsana.

Having kept both the hands under both the thighs, with the body straight, when one sits calmly in this posture, it is called Swastika.

22.) savye dakṣhiṇa-ghulkaṃ tu pṛṣhṭha-pārśve niyojayet ǀ dakṣhiṇeǀapi tathā savy-aṃ ghomukhaṃ ghomukhākṛtiḥ

Gomukha-âsana.

Placing the right ankle on the left side and the left ankle on the right side, makes Gomukha-âsana, having the appearance of a cow.

23.) ekaṃ pādaṃ tathaikasminvinyaseduruṇi sthiram | itarasmiṃstathā choruṃ vīrāsanamitīritam

Vîrâsana.

One foot is to be placed on the thigh of the opposite side; and so also the other foot on the opposite thigh. This is called Vîrâsana.

24.) ghudaṃ nirudhya ghulphābhyāṃ vyutkrameṇa samāhitaḥ | kūrmāsanaṃ bhavedetaditi yogha-vido viduḥ

Kurmâsana.

Placing the right ankle on the left side of anus, and the left ankle on the right side of it, makes what the Yogîs call Kûrma-âsana.

25.) padmāsanaṃ tu saṃsthāpya jānūrvorantare karau | niveśya bhūmau saṃsthāpya vyomasthaṃ kukkuṭāsanam

Kukkuta-âsana.

*Taking the posture of Padma-âsana and carrying the
hands under the thighs, when the Yogî raises himself
above the ground, with his palms resting on the ground,
it becomes Kukkuta-âsana.*

26.) kukkuṭāsana-bandha-stho dorbhyāṃ sambadya kandharām | bhavedkūrmavaduttāna etaduttāna-kūrmakam

Uttâna Kûrma-âsana.

*Having assumed Kukkuta-âsana, when one grasps his
neck by crossing his hands behind his head, and lies
in this posture with his back touching the ground, it
becomes Uttâna Kûrma-âsana, from its appearance like
that of a tortoise.*

27.) pādāngghuṣhṭhau tu pāṇibhyāṃ ghṛhītvā śravaṇāvadhi | dhanurākarṣhaṇaṃ kuryāddhanur-āsanamuchyate

Dhanura-âsana.

*Having caught the toes of the feet with both the hands
and carried them to the ears by drawing the body like a
bow, it becomes Dhanura âsana.*

28+29.) vāmoru-mūlārpita-dakṣha-pādaṃ
jānorbahirveṣhṭita-vāma-pādam | praghṛhya
tiṣhṭhetparivartitānggghaḥ śrī-matysanāthodi-
tamāsanaṃ syāt

**matsyendra-pīṭhaṃ jaṭhara-pradīptiṃ
prachaṇḍa-rughmaṇḍala-khaṇḍanāstram |
abhyāsataḥ kuṇḍalinī-prabodhaṃ chandra-st-
hiratvaṃ cha dadāti puṃsām**

Matsyendrâsana.

*Having placed the right foot at the root of the left thigh,
let the toe be grasped with the right hand passing over
the back, and having placed the left foot on the right
thigh at its root, let it be grasped with the left hand
passing behind the back. This is the âsana, as explained
by Śri Matsyanâtha.*

*It increases appetite and is an instrument for destroy-
ing the group of the most deadly diseases. Its practice
awakens the Kundalinî, stops the nectar shedding from
the moon in people.*

**30.) prasārya pādau bhuvi daṇḍa-rūpau dor-
bhyāṃ padāghra-dvitayaṃ ghṛhītvā | jānūpa-
rinyasta-lalāṭa-deśo vasedidaṃ paśchimatā-
namāhuḥ**

Paśchima Tâna.

*Having stretched the feet on the ground, like a stick, and
having grasped the toes of both the feet with both the
hands, when one sits with his forehead resting on the
thighs, it is called Paśchima Tâna.*

**31.) iti paśchimatānamāsanāghryaṃ pavanaṃ
paśchima-vāhinaṃ karoti | udayaṃ jaṭharā-
nalasya kuryād udare kārśyamaroghatāṃ cha
puṃsām**

*This Paśchima Tâna carries the air from the front to the
back part of the body (i.e., to the sushumna). It kindles
gastric fire, reduces obesity and cures all diseases of men.*

**32.) dharāmavaṣhṭabhya kara-dvayena
tat-kūrpara-sthāpita-nābhi-pārśvaḥ | uchchā-
sano daṇḍavadutthitaḥ khe māyūrametatpra-
vadanti pīṭham**

Mayûra-âsana.

*Place the palms of both the hands on the ground, and
place the navel on both the elbows and balancing thus,
the body should be stretched backward like a stick. This
is called Mayûra-âsana.*

**33.) harati sakala-roghānāśu ghulmodarādīn
abhibhavati cha doṣhānāsanam śrī-mayūram
I bahu kadaśana-bhuktam bhasma kuryā-
daśeṣham janayati jaṭharāghnim jārayet-
kāla-kūṭam**

*This Âsana soon destroys all diseases, and removes
abdominal disorders, and also those arising from irregu-
larities of phlegm, bile and wind, digests unwholesome
food taken in excess, increases appetite and destroys the
most deadly poison.*

**34.) uttānam śabavadbhūmau śayanam
tachchavāsanam I śavāsanam śrānti-haram
chitta-viśrānti-kārakam**

Śava-âsana.

*Lying down on the ground, like a corpse, is called Śa-
va-âsana. It removes fatigue and gives rest to the mind.*

**35.) chaturaśītyāsanāni śivena kathitāni cha I
tebhyaśchatuṣhkamādāya sārabhūtam bravī-
myaham**

*Śiva taught 84 âsanas. Of these the first four being essen-
tial ones, I am going to explain them here.*

36.) siddhaṃ padmaṃ tathā siṃhaṃ bhadraṃ veti chatuṣhṭayam । śreṣhṭham tatrāpi cha sukhe tiṣhṭhetsiddhāsane sadā

These four are: The Siddha, Padma, Sinha and Bhadra. Even of these, the Siddha-âsana, being very comfortable, one should always practise it.

37.) atha siddhāsanam yoni-sthānakamangghri-mūla-ghaṭitaṃ kṛtvā dṛḍhaṃ vinyaset meṇḍhre pādamathaikame- va hṛdaye kṛtvā hanuṃ susthiram । sthāṇuḥ saṃyamitendriyo|achala-dṛśā paśyedbh- ruvorantaraṃ hyetanmokṣha-kapāṭa-bhe- da-janakaṃ siddhāsanaṃ prochyate

The Siddhâsana.

Press firmly the heel of the left foot against the peri- neum, and the right heel above the male organ. With the chin pressing on the chest, one should sit calmly, having restrained the senses, and gaze steadily the space between the eyebrows. This is called the Siddha Âsana, the opener of the door of salvation.

38.) meṇḍhrādupari vinyasya savyaṃ ghulphaṃ tathopari । ghulphāntaraṃ cha nikṣhipya siddhāsanamidaṃ bhavet

This Siddhâsana is performed also by placing the left heel on Medhra (above the male organ), and then placing the right one on it.

39.) etatsiddhāsanaṃ prāhuranye vajrāsanaṃ viduḥ I muktāsanaṃ vadantyeke prāhurghuptāsanaṃ pare

Some call this Siddhâsana, some Vajrâsana. Others call it Mukta Âsana or Gupta Âsana.

40.) syameṣhviva mitāhāramahiṃsā niyameṣhviva I mukhyaṃ sarvāsaneṣhvekaṃ siddhāḥ siddhāsanaṃ viduḥ

Just as sparing food is among Yamas, and Ahimsâ among the Niyamas, so is Siddhâsana called by adepts the chief of all the âsanas.

41.) chaturaśīti-pītheshu siddhameva sadābhyaset I dvāsaptati-sahasrānām nādīnām mala-śodhanam

Out of the 84 Âsanas Siddhâsana should always be practised, because it cleanses the impurities of 72,000 nâdîs.

42.) ātma-dhyāyī mitāhārī yāvaddvādaśa-vat-saram I sadā siddhāsanābhyāsādyoghī nishpattimāpnuyāt

By contemplating on oneself, by eating sparingly, and by practising Siddhâsana for 12 years, the Yogî obtains success.

43.) kimanyairbahubhiḥ pīṭhaiḥ siddhe sidd-hāsane sati I prāṇānile sāvadhāne baddhe kevala-kumbhake I utpadyate nirāyāsātsvay-amevonmanī kalā

Other postures are of no use, when success has been achieved in Siddhâsana, and Prâna Vâyû becomes calm and restrained by Kevala Kumbhaka.

44.) tathaikāsminneva drdhe siddhe siddhā-sane sati I bandha-trayamanāyāsātsvaya-mevopajāyate

Success in one Siddhâsana alone becoming firmly esta-blished, one gets Unmanî at once, and the three bonds (Bandhas) are accomplished of themselves.

45.) nāsanaṃ siddha-sadṛśaṃ na kumbhaḥ kevalopamaḥ I na khecharī-samā mudrā na nāda-sadṛśo layaḥ

There is no Âsana like the Siddhâsana and no Kumbha-ka like the Kevala. There is no mudrâ like the Khechari and no laya like the Nâda (Anâhata Nâda.)

46.) atha padmāsanam

vāmorūpari dakṣhiṇaṃ cha charaṇaṃ

saṃsthāpya vāmaṃ tathā dakṣhorūpa-

ri paśchimena vidhinā dhṛtvā karābhyāṃ

dṛḍham I angghuṣhṭhau hṛdaye nidhāya

chibukaṃnāsāghramālokayet etadvyād-

hi-vināśa-kāri yamināṃ padmāsanaṃ prochy-

ate

The Padmâsana.

Place the right foot on the left thigh and the left foot on the right thigh, and grasp the toes with the hands crossed over the back. Press the chin against the chest and gaze on the tip of the nose. This is called the Padmâsana, the destroyer of the diseases of the Yamîs.

47.) uttānau charaṇau kṛtvā ūru-saṃsthau

prayatnataḥ I ūru-madhye tathottānau pāṇī

kṛtvā tato dṛśau

Place the feet on the thighs, with the soles upwards, and place the hands on the thighs, with the palms upwards.

48.) nāsāghre vinyasedrājad-anta-mūle tu jihvayā | uttambhya chibukam vakṣhasyutt-hāpy pavanam śanaiḥ

Gaze on the tip of the nose, keeping the tongue pressed against the root of the teeth of the upper jaw, and the chin against the chest, and raise the air up slowly, i.e., pull the apâna-vâyû gently upwards.

49.) idam padmāsanam proktam sarva-vyād-hi-vināśanam | durlabham yena kenāpi dhīmatā labhyate bhuvi

This is called the Padmâsana, the destroyer of all dise-ases. It is difficult of attainment by everybody, but can be learnt by intelligent people in this world.

50.) kṛtvā sampuṭitau karau dṛḍhataram badd-hvā tu padmamāsanam ghāḍham vakṣhasi sannidhāya chibukam dhyāyamścha tach-chetasi | vāram vāramapānamūrdhvamanilam protsārayanpūritam nyañchanprāṇamupaiti bodhamatulam śakti-prabhāvānnaraḥ

Having kept both the hands together in the lap, perfor-ming the Padmâsana firmly, keeping the chin Fixed to the chest and contemplating on Him in the mind, by

drawing the apâna-vâyû up (performing Mûla Bandha)
and pushing down the air after inhaling it, joining thus
the prâna and apâna in the navel, one gets the highest
intelligence by awakening the śakti (kundalinî) thus.

NB.—When Apâna Vâyû is drawn gently up and after
filling in the lungs with the air from outside, the prâna is
forced down by and by so as to join both of them in the
navel, they both enter then the Kundalinî and, reaching
the Brahma randhra (the great hole), they make the
mind calm. Then the mind can contemplate on the na-
ture of the âtmana and can enjoy the highest bliss.

51.) padmāsane sthito yoghī nāḍī-dvāreṇa pūritam mārutaṃ dhārayedyastu sa mukto nātra saṃśayaḥ

The Yogî who, sitting with Padmâsana, can control bre-
athing, there is no doubt, is free from bondage.

52.) atha siṃhāsanam
ghulphau cha vṛṣhaṇasyādhaḥ sīvantyāḥ pārśvayoḥ kṣhipet I dakṣhiṇe savya-ghulp-ham tu dakṣha- ghulpham tu savyake

The Simhâsana.

*Press the heels on both sides of the seam of Perineum, in
such a way that the left heel touches the right side and
the right heel touches the left side of it.*

53.) hastau tu jānvoḥ saṃsthāpya svāngg-hulīḥ sam-prasārya cha | vyātta-vakto nirīkṣ-heta nāsāgh-raṃ susamāhitaḥ

*Place the hands on the thighs, with stretched fingers,
and keeping the mouth open and the mind collected,
gaze on the tip of the nose.*

54.) siṃhāsanaṃ bhavedetatpūjitaṃ yog-hi-pungghavaiḥ | bandha-tritaya-sandhānaṃ kurute chāsanottamam

*This is Simhâsana, held sacred by the best of Yogîs. This
excellent Âsana effects the completion of the three Band-
has (The Mûlabandha, Kantha or Jâlandhar Bandha
and Uddiyâna Bandha).*

55+56.) atha bhadrāsanam
ghulphau cha vṛṣhaṇasyādhaḥ sīvantyāḥ pārśvayoḥ kṣhipte | savya-ghulphaṃ tathā savye dakṣha-ghulphaṃ tu dakṣhiṇe

pārśva-pādau cha pāṇibhyāṃ dṛḍhaṃ baddh-vā suniśchalam | bhadrāsanaṃ bhavedetats-

arva-vyādhi-vināśanam | ghorakṣhāsanami-
tyāhuridaṃ vai siddha-yoghinaḥ

The Bhadrâsana.

*Place the heels on either side of the seam of the Peri-
neum, keeping the left heel on the left side and the right
one on the right side, hold the feet firmly joined to one
another with both the hands. This Bhadrâsana is the
destroyer of all the diseases.*

57.) evamāsana-bandheṣhu yoghīndro vig-
hata-śramaḥ | abhyasennāḍikā-śuddhiṃ
mudrādi-pavanī-kriyām

*The expert Yogîs call this Gorakśa âsana. By sitting with
this âsana, the Yogî gets rid of fatigue.*

58.) āsanaṃ kumbhakaṃ chitraṃ mudrākhy-
aṃ karaṇaṃ tathā | atha nādānusandhāna-
mabhyāsānukramo haṭhe

*The Nâdis should be cleansed of their impurities by
performing the mudrâs, etc. (which are the practices
relating to the air). Âsanas, Kumbhakas and various
curious mûdrâs.*

**59.) brahmachārī mitāhārī tyāghī yog-
ha-parāyaṇaḥ | abdādūrdhvaṃ bhavedsidd-
ho nātra kāryā vichāraṇā**

*By regular and close attention to Nâda (anâhata nâda)
in Hatha Yoga, a Brahmachari, sparing in diet, unat-
tached to objects of enjoyment, and devoted to Yoga,
gains success, no doubt, within a year.*

**60.) susnighdha-madhurāhāraścha-
turthāṃśa-vivarjitaḥ | bhujyate śi-
va-samprītyai mitāharaḥ sa uchyate**

*Abstemious feeding is that in which ¾ of hunger is sa-
tisfied with food, well cooked with ghee and sweets, and
eaten with the offering of it to Śiva.*

**61.) kaṭvāmla-tīkṣhṇa-lavaṇoṣhṇa-harīta-śāka-
sauvīra-taila-tila-sarṣhapa-madya-matsyān
| ājādi-māṃsa-dadhi-takra-kulatthakola-
piṇyāka-hingghu-laśunādyamapathyamāhuḥ**

Foods injurious to a Yogî.

*Bitter, sour, saltish, hot, green vegetables, fermented,
oily, mixed with til seed, rape seed, intoxicating liquors,
fish, meat, curds, chhaasa pulses, plums, oil-cake, asafo-
etida (hînga), garlic, onion, etc. should not be eaten.*

**62.) sbhojanamahitaṃ vidyātpuna-
rasyoṣhṇī-kṛtaṃ rūkṣham | atilavaṇamam-
la-yuktaṃ kadaśana-śākotkaṃ varjyam**

*Food heated again, dry, having too much salt, sour, mi-
nor grains, and vegetables that cause burning sensation,
should not be eaten, Fire, women, travelling, etc., should
be avoided.*

**63.) vahni-strī-pathi-sevānāmādau varja-
namācharet**

*As said by Goraksa, one should keep aloof from the
society of the evil-minded, fire, women, travelling, early
morning bath, fasting, and all kinds of bodily exertion.*

**64.) tathā hi ghorakṣha-vachanam varjayed-
durjana-prāntaṃ vahni-strī-pathi-sevanam
| prātaḥ-snānopavāsādi kāya-kleśa-vidhiṃ
tathā**

*Wheat, rice, barley, shâstik (a kind of rice), good corns,
milk, ghee, sugar, butter, sugarcandy, honey, dried ging-
er, Parwal (a vegetable) the five vegetables, moong, pure
water, these are very beneficial to those who practise
Yoga.*

65.) hodhūma-śāli-yava-ṣhāṣhṭika-śobhanān-nam kṣhīrājya-khaṇḍa-navanīta-sidd-hā-madhūni | śuṇṭhī-paṭola-kaphalādi-ka-pañcha-śākaṃ mudghādi-divyamudakaṃ cha yamīndra-pathyam

A Yogî should eat tonics (things giving strength), well sweetened, greasy (made with ghee), milk, butter, etc., which may increase humors of the body, according to his desire.

66.) puṣhṭaṃ sumadhuraṃ snighdhaṃ ghavy-am dhātu-prapoṣhaṇam | manobhilaṣhitaṃ yoghyaṃ yoghī bhojanamācharet

Whether young, old or too old, sick or lean, one who discards laziness, gets success if he practises Yoga.

67.) yuvo vṛddho|ativṛddho vā vyādhito dur-balo|api vā | abhyāsātsiddhimāpnoti sar-va-yogheṣhvatandritaḥ

Success comes to him who is engaged in the practice. How can one get success without practice; for by merely reading books on Yoga, one can never get success.

68.) kriyā-yuktasya siddhiḥ syādakriyasya

katham bhavet | na śāstra-pāṭha-mātreṇa yogha-siddhiḥ prajāyate

Success cannot be attained by adopting a particular dress (Vesa). It cannot be gained by telling tales. Practice alone is the means to success. This is true, there is no doubt.

69+70.) na veṣha-dhāraṇam siddheḥ kāraṇam na cha tat-kathā | kriyaiva kāraṇam siddheḥ satyametanna saṃśayaḥ

pīṭhāni kumbhakāśchitrā divyāni karaṇāni cha | sarvāṇyapi haṭhābhyāse rāja-yog-ha-phalāvadhi

Âsanas (postures), various Kumbhakas, and other divine means, all should be practised in the practice of Hatha Yoga, till the fruit—Râja Yoga—is obtained.

iti haṭha-pradīpikāyāṃ prathamopadeśaḥ

End of chapter 1st, on the method of forming the Âsa-nas.

Chapter 2

Pranayamas

Dvitīyopadeśah

1.) athāsane dṛdhe yoghī vaśī hita-mitāśanaḥ | ghurūpadiṣhṭa-mārgheṇa prāṇāyāmānsam-abhyaset

Posture becoming established, a Yogî, master of himself, eating salutary and moderate food, should practise Prânâyâma, as instructed by his guru.

2.) chale vāte chalaṃ chittam niśchale niśchalaṃ bhavet ‖ yoghī sthāṇutvamāpnoti tato vāyuṃ nirodhayet

Respiration being disturbed, the mind becomes disturbed. By restraining respiration, the Yogî gets steadiness of mind.

3.) yāvadvāyuḥ sthito dehe tāvajjīvanamuchy-ate | maraṇaṃ tasya niṣhkrāntistato vāyuṃ nirodhayet

So long as the (breathing) air stays in the body, it is called life. Death consists in the passing out of the (breathing) air. It is, therefore, necessary to restrain the breath.

**4.) malākalāsu nāḍīṣhu māruto naiva mad-
hyaghaḥ | kathaṃ syādunmanībhāvaḥ
kārya-siddhiḥ kathaṃ bhavet**

*The breath does not pass through the middle channel
(susumnâ), owing to the impurities of the nâdîs. How
can then success be attained, and how can there be the
unmanî avasthâ.*

**5.) śuddhameti yadā sarvaṃ nāḍī-chakraṃ
malākulam | tadaiva jāyate yoghī
prāṇa-saṃghrahaṇe kṣhamaḥ**

*When the whole system of nâdîs which is full of impuri-
ties, is cleaned, then the Yogî becomes able to control the
Prâna.*

**6.) prāṇāyāmaṃ tataḥ kuryānnityaṃ sātt-
vikayā dhiyā | yathā suṣhumṇā-nāḍīsthā
malāḥ śuddhiṃ prayānti cha**

*Therefore, Prânâyâma should be performed daily with
sâtwika buddhi (intellect free from raja and tama or
activity and sloth), in order to drive out the impurities of
the susumnâ.*

7+8.) baddha-padmāsano yoghī prāṇaṃ

chandreṇa pūrayet | dhārayitvā yathā-śakti
bhūyaḥ sūryeṇa rechayet

prāṇaṃ sūryeṇa chākṛṣhya pūrayedudaraṃ
śanaiḥ | vidhivatkumbhakaṃ kṛtvā punaśch-
andreṇa rechayet

Method of performing Prânâyâma.

*Sitting in the Padmâsana posture the Yogî should fill
in the air through the left nostril (closing the right
one); and, keeping it confined according to one's ability,
it should be expelled slowly through the sûrya (right
nostril). Then, drawing in the air through the sûrya
(right nostril) slowly, the belly should be filled, and after
performing Kumbhaka as before, it should be expelled
slowly through the chandra (left nostril).*

**9.) yena tyajettena pītvā dhārayedatirodha-
taḥ | rechayechcha tato|anyena śanaireva na
veghataḥ**

*Inhaling thus through the one, through which it was
expelled, and having restrained it there, till possible,
it should be exhaled through the other, slowly and not
forcibly.*

10.) prāṇaṃ chediḍayā pibenniyamitaṃ bhūyo I anyathā rechayet pītvā pingghalayā samīraṇamatho baddhvā tyajedvāmayā I sūrya-chandramasoranena vidhinābhyāsaṃ sadā tanvatāṃ śuddhā nāḍi-ghaṇā bhavanti yaminām māsa-trayādūrdhvataḥ

If the air be inhaled through the left nostril, it should be expelled again through the other, and filling it through the right nostril, confining it there, it should be expelled through the left nostril. By practising in this way, through the right and the left nostrils alternately, the whole of the collection of the nâdîs of the yamîs (practisers) becomes clean, i.e., free from impurities, after 3 months and over.

11.) prātarmadhyandine sāyamardha-rātre cha kumbhakān I śanairaśīti-paryantaṃ chatur-vāraṃ samabhyaset

Kumbhakas should be performed gradually 4 times during day and night, i.e., (morning, noon, evening and midnight), till the number of Kumbhakas for one time is 80 and for day and night together it is 320.

12.) kanīyasi bhavedsveda kampo bhavati madhyame I uttame sthānamāpnoti tato vāyum nibandhayet

In the beginning there is perspiration, in the middle stage there is quivering, and in the last or the 3rd stage one obtains steadiness; and then the breath should be made steady or motionless.

13.) jalena śrama-jātena ghātra-marda-namācharet | dṛḍhatā laghutā chaiva tena ghātrasya jāyate

The perspiration exuding from exertion of practice should be rubbed into the body (and not wiped), as by so doing the body becomes strong.

14.) abhyāsa-kāle prathame śastaṃ kṣhīrājya-bhojanam | tato|abhyāse dṛḍhībhū-te na tādṛṅg-niyama-ghrahaḥ

During the first stage of practice the food consisting of milk and ghee is wholesome. When the practice becomes established, no such restriction is necessary.

15.) yathā siṃho ghajo vyāghro bhavedvaśy-aḥ śanaiḥ śanaiḥ | tathaiva sevito vāyurany-athā hanti sādhakam

Just as lions, elephants and tigers are controlled by and by, so the breath is controlled by slow degrees, otherwise (i.e., by being hasty or using too much force) it kills the practiser himself.

16.) prāṇāyāmena yuktena sarva-rog-ha-kṣhayo bhavet | ayuktābhyāsa-yoghena sarva-rogha-samudghamaḥ

When Prânayama, etc., are performed properly, they eradicate all diseases; but an improper practice generates diseases.

17.) hikkā śvāsaścha kāsaścha śi-raḥ-karṇākṣhi-vedanāḥ | bhavanti vividhāḥ roghāḥ pavanasya prakopataḥ*

Hiccough, asthma, cough, pain in the head, the ears, and the eyes; these and other various kinds of diseases are generated by the disturbance of the breath.

18.) yuktaṃ yuktaṃ tyajedvāyuṃ yuktaṃ yuktaṃ cha pūrayet | yuktaṃ yuktaṃ cha badhnīyādevaṃ siddhimavāpnuyāt

The air should be expelled with proper tact and should be filled in skilfully; and when it has been kept confined properly it brings success.

NB.—The above caution is necessary to warn the aspirants against omitting any instruction; and, in their zeal to gain success or siddhis early, to begin the practice, either by using too much force in filling in, confining and expelling the air, or by omitting any instructions, it may cause unnecessary pressure on their ears, eyes, &c,, and cause pain. Every word in the instructions is full of meaning and is necessarily used in the slokas, and should be followed very carefully and with due attention. Thus there will be nothing to fear whatsoever. We are inhaling and exhaling the air throughout our lives without any sort of danger, and Prânayama being only a regular form of it, there should be no cause to fear.

19.) yadā tu nāḍī-śuddhiḥ syāttathā chihnāni bāhyataḥ I kāyasya kṛśatā kāntistadā jāyate niśchitam

When the nâdîs become free from impurities, and there appear the outward signs of success, such as lean body and glowing colour, then one should feel certain of success.

20.) yatheṣhṭaṃ dhāraṇaṃ vāyoranalasya pradīpanam I nādābhivyaktirāroghyaṃ jāyate nāḍi-śodhanāt

By removing the impurities, the air can be restrained, according to one's wish and the appetite is increased, the divine sound is awakened, and the body becomes healthy.

21.) meda-śleṣhmādhikaḥ pūrvaṃ ṣhaṭ-karmāṇi samācharet | anyastu nācharettāni doṣhāṇāṃ samabhāvataḥ

If there be excess of fat or phlegm in the body, the six kinds of kriyâs (duties) should be performed first. But others, not suffering from the excess of these, should not perform them.

22.) dhautirbastistathā netistrāṭakaṃ nau-likaṃ tathā | kapāla-bhātiśchaitāni ṣhaṭ-karmāṇi prachakṣhate

The six kinds of duties are: Dhauti, Basti, Neti, Trâtaka, Nauti and Kapâla Bhâti. These are called the six actions.

23.) karma ṣhaṭkamidaṃ ghopyaṃ ghaṭa-śod-hana-kārakam | vichitra-ghuṇa-sandhāya pūjyate yoghi-pungghavaiḥ

These six kinds of actions which cleanse the body should be kept secret. They produce extraordinary attributes and are performed with earnestness by the best of Yogîs.

**24.) tatra dhautiḥ
chatur-angghula-vistāraṃ has-
ta-pañcha-daśāyatam | ghurūpadiṣhṭa-mārg-
heṇa siktaṃ vastraṃ śanairghraset | punaḥ
pratyāharechchaitaduditaṃ dhauti-karma tat**

The Dhauti.

*A strip of cloth, about 3 inches wide and 15 cubits long,
is pushed in (swallowed), when moist with warm water,
through the passage shown by the guru, and is taken out
again. This is called Dhauti Karma.*

*NB.—The strip should be moistened with a little warm
water, and the end should be held with the teeth. It is
swallowed slowly, little by little; thus, first day 1 cubit,
2nd day 2 cubits, 3rd day 3 cubits, and so on. After
swallowing it the stomach should be given a good, round
motion from left to right, and then it should be taken
out slowly and gently.*

**25.) kāsa-śvāsa-plīha-kuṣhṭhaṃ kapharog-
hāścha viṃśatiḥ | dhauti-karma-prabhāveṇa
prayāntyeva na saṃśayaḥ**

*There is no doubt, that cough, asthma, enlargement
of the spleen, leprosy, and 20 kinds of diseases born of
phlegm, disappear by the practice of Dhauti Karma.*

26.) atha bastiḥ
nābhi-daghna-jale pāyau nyasta-nālotkaṭās-
anaḥ | ādhārākuñchanaṃ kuryātkṣhālanaṃ
basti-karma tat

The Basti.

Squatting in navel-deep water, and introducing a six in-
ches long, smooth piece of ½ an inch diameter pipe, open
at both ends, half inside the anus; it (anus) should he
drawn up (contracted) and then expelled. This washing
is called the Basti Karma.

27.) ghulma-plīhodaraṃ chāpi vāta-pitta-kap-
hodbhavāḥ | basti-karma-prabhāveṇa kṣhīy-
ante sakalāmayāḥ

By practising this Basti Karma, colic, enlarged spleen,
and dropsy, arising from the disorders of Vâta (air),
pitta (bile) and kapha (phlegm), are all cured.

28.) dhāntvadriyāntaḥ-karaṇa-prasādaṃ
dadhāchcha kāntiṃ dahana-pradīptam |
aśeṣha-doṣhopachayaṃ nihanyād abhyasy-
amānaṃ jala-basti-karma

By practising Basti with water, the Dhâtâs, the Indriyas

*and the mind become calm. It gives glow and tone to
the body and increases the appetite. All the disorders
disappear.*

**29.) atha netiḥ
sūtraṃ vitasti-susnighdhaṃ nāsānāle pra-
veśayet ǀ mukhānnirghamayechchaiṣhā
netiḥ siddhairnighadyate**

The Neti.

*A cord made of threads and about six inches long,
should be passed through the passage of the nose and
the end taken out in the mouth. This is called by adepts
the Neti Karma.*

**30.) kapāla-śodhinī chaiva divya-dṛṣhṭi-
pradāyinī ǀ jatrūrdhva-jāta-roghaughaṃ
netirāśu nihanti cha**

*The Neti is the cleaner of the brain and giver of divine
sight. It soon destroys all the diseases of the cervical and
scapular regions.*

**31.) atha trāṭakam
nirīkṣhenniśchala-dṛśā sūkṣhma-lakṣhyaṃ
samāhitaḥ ǀ aśru-sampāta-paryantamāchāry-
aistrāṭakaṃ smṛtam**

The Trâtaka.

*Being calm, one should gaze steadily at a small mark,
till eyes are filled with tears. This is called Trataka by
âchâryas.*

32.) mochanaṃ netra-roghāṇāṃ tandādrīṇāṃ kapāṭakam I yatnatastrāṭakaṃ ghopyaṃ yathā hāṭaka-peṭakam

*Trâtaka destroys the eye diseases and removes sloth,
etc. It should be kept secret very carefully, like a box of
jewellery.*

33.) atha nauliḥ amandāvarta-veghena tundaṃ savyāpasavya-taḥ I natāṃso bhrāmayedeṣhā nauliḥ sidd-haiḥ praśasyate

The Nauli.

*Sitting on the toes with heels raised above the ground,
and the palms resting on the ground, and in this bent
posture the belly is moved forcibly from left to right just,
as in vomiting. This is called by adepts the Nauli Karma.*

**34.) mandāghni-sandīpana-pāchanādi-sand-
hāpikānanda-karī sadaiva | aśeṣha-doṣha-
maya-śoṣhaṇī cha haṭha-kriyā mauliriyaṃ
cha nauliḥ**

*It removes dyspepsia, increases appetite and digestion,
and is like the goddess of creation, and causes happiness.
It dries up all the disorders. This Nauli is an excellent
exercise in Hatha Yoga.*

**35.) atha kapālabhātiḥ
bhastrāvalloha-kārasya recha-pūrau sasam-
bhramau | kapālabhātirvikhyātā kapha-
doṣha-viśoṣhaṇī**

The Kapâla Bhâti.

*When inhalation and exhalation are performed very
quickly, like a pair of bellows of a blacksmith, it dries
up all the disorders from the excess of phlegm, and is
known as Kapâla Bhâti.*

**36.) ṣhaṭ-karma-nirghata-sthaulya-kap-
ha-doṣha-malādikaḥ | prāṇāyāmaṃ tataḥ
kuryādanāyāsena siddhyati**

When Prânâyâma is performed after getting rid of

obesity born of the defects phlegm, by the performance
of the six duties, it easily brings success.

37.) prāṇāyāmaireva sarve praśuṣhyanti malā iti | āchāryāṇāṃ tu keṣhāṃchidanyatkarma na saṃmatam

Some âchâryâs (teachers) do not advocate any other
practice, being of opinion that all the impurities are
dried up by the practice of Prânâyâma.

38.) atha ghaja-karaṇī udara-ghata-padārthamudvamanti pavana-mapānamudīrya kaṇṭha-nāle | krama-pa-richaya-vaśya-nāḍi-chakrā ghaja-karaṇīti nighadyate haṭhajñaiḥ

Gaja Karani.

By carrying the Apâna Vâyû up to the throat, the food,
etc., in the stomach are vomited. By degrees, the system
of Nâdîs (Śankhinî) becomes known. This is called in
Hatha as Gaja Karani.

39.) brahmādayo|api tridaśāḥ pavanābhyā-sa-tatparāḥ | abhūvannantaka-bhyāttasmāt-pavanamabhyaset

*Brahmâ, and other Devas were always engaged in
the exercise of Prânâyâma, and, by means of it, got
rid of the fear of death. Therefore, one should practise
prânâyâma regularly.*

40.) yāvadbaddho marud-deśe yāvachchit-
tam nirākulam I yāvaddṛṣhṭirbhruvormadhye
tāvatkāla-bhayaṃ kutaḥ

*So long as the breath is restrained in the body, so long as
the mind is undisturbed, and so long as the gaze is fixed
between the eyebrows, there is no fear from Death.*

41.) vidhivatprāṇa-saṃyāmairnāḍī-chakre
viśodhite I suṣhumṇā-vadanaṃ bhittvā suk-
hādviśati mārutaḥ

*When the system of Nâdis becomes clear of the impu-
rities by properly controlling the prâna, then the air,
piercing the entrance of the Suśumnâ, enters it easily.*

42.) atha manonmanī
mārute madhya-saṃchāre manaḥ-sthairy-
am prajāyate I yo manaḥ-susthirī-bhāvaḥ
saivāvasthā manonmanī

Manomanî.

Steadiness of mind comes when the air moves Freely in the middle. That is the manonmanî condition, which is attained when the mind becomes calm.

43.) tat-siddhaye vidhānajñāśchitrānkurvanti kumbhakān l vichitra kumbhakābhyāsādvichitrāṃ siddhimāpnuyāt

To accomplish it, various Kumbhakas are performed by those who are expert in the methods; for, by the practice of different Kumbhakas, wonderful success is attained.

44.) atha kumbhaka-bhedāḥ sūrya-bhedanamujjāyī sītkārī śītalī tathā l bhastrikā bhrāmarī mūrchchā plāvinītyaṣhṭa-kumbhakāḥ

Different hinds of Kumbhakas. Kumbhakas are of eight kinds, viz., Sûrya Bhedan, Ujjâyî, Sîtkarî, Sîtalî, Bhastrikâ, Bhrâmarî, Mûrchhâ, and Plâvinî.

45.) pūrakānte tu kartavyo bandho jālandharābhidhaḥ l kumbhakānte rechakādau kartavyastūḍḍiyānakaḥ

At the end of Pûraka, Jâlandhara Bandha should be performed, and at the end of Kumbhaka, and at the beginning of Rechaka, Uddiyâna Bandha should be performed.

NB.—Pûraka is filling in of the air from outside.

Kumbhaka is the keeping the air confined inside. Rechaka is expelling the confined air. The instructions for Puraka, Kumbhaka and Rechaka will be found at their proper place and should he carefully followed.

46.) adhastātkuñchanenāśu kaṇṭha-sang-kochane kṛte I madhye paśchima-tānena syātprāṇo brahma-nāḍighaḥ

By drawing up from below (Mûla Bandha) and contracting the throat (Jâlandhara Bandha) and by pulling back the middle of the front portion of the body (i.e., belly), the Prâna goes to the Brahma Nâdî (Susumnâ).

The middle hole, through the vertebral column, through which the spinal cord passes, is called the Susumnâ Nâdî of the Yogîs. The two other sympathetic cords, one on each aide of the spinal cord, are called the Idâ and the Pingalâ Nâdîs. These will be described later on.

**47.) āpānamūrdhvamutthāpya prāṇaṃ
kaṇṭhādadho nayet I yoghī jarā-vimuktaḥ
sanṣhoḍaśābda-vayā bhavet**

*By pulling up the Apâna Vâyu and by forcing the Prâna
Vâyu down the throat, the Yogî, liberated from old age,
becomes young, as it were 16 years old.*

Note.

*The seat of the Prâna is the heart; of the Apâna anus; of
the Samâna the region about the navel; of the Udâna the
throat; while the Vyâna moves throughout the body.*

**48.) atha sūrya-bhedanam
āsane sukhade yoghī baddhvā chaivāsanaṃ
tataḥ I dakṣha-nāḍyā samākṛṣhya bahiḥst-
haṃ pavanaṃ śanaiḥ**

Sûrya Bhedana.

*Taking any comfortable posture and performing the
âsana, the Yogî should draw in the air slowly, through
the right nostril.*

**49.) ākeśādānakhāghrāchcha nirodhāvad-
hi kumbhayet I tataḥ śanaiḥ savya-nāḍyā
rechayetpavanaṃ śanaiḥ**

Then it should be confined within, so that it fills from the nails to the tips of the hair, and then let out through the left nostril slowly.

Note. This is to be done alternately with both the nostrils, drawing in through the one, expelling through the other, and vice versa.

50.) kapāla-śodhanaṃ vāta-doṣha-ghnaṃ kṛmi-doṣha-hṛt I punaḥ punaridaṃ kāryaṃ sūrya-bhedanamuttamam

This excellent Sûrya Bhedana cleanses the forehead (frontal sinuses), destroys the disorders of Vâta, and removes the worms, and, therefore, it should be performed again and again.

Note.

Translation: I am going to describe the procedure of the practice of Yoga, in order that Yogîs may succeed. A wise man should leave his bed in the Usâ Kâla (i.e. at the peep of dawn or 4 o'clock) in the morning. 1.

Remembering his guru over his head, and his desired deity in his heart, after answering the calls of nature, and cleaning his mouth, he should apply Bhasma (ashes). 2.

In a clean spot, clean room and charming ground, he should spread a soft âsana (cloth for sitting on). Having seated on it and remembering, in his mind his guru and his God. 3.

Having extolled the place and the time and taking up the vow thus: 'To day by the grace of God, I will perform Prânâyâmas with âsanas for gaining samâdhi (trance) and its fruits.' He should salute the infinite Deva, Lord of the Nâgas, to ensure success in the âsanas (postures). 4.

Salutation to the Lord of the Nâgas, who is adorned with thousands of heads, set with brilliant jewels (manis), and who has sustained the whole universe, nourishes it, and is infinite. After this he should begin his exercise of âsanas and when fatigued, he should practise Śava âsana. Should there be no fatigue, he should not practise it. 5.

Before Kumbhaka, he should perform Viparîta Karnî mudrâ, in order that he may be able to perform Jâlandhar bandha comfortably. 6.

Sipping a little water, he should begin the exercise of Prânâyâma, after saluting Yogindras, as described in the Karma Parana, in the words of Śiva. 7.

Such as "Saluting Yogindras and their disciples and gurû Vinâyaka, the Yogî should unite with me with composed mind." 8.

While practising, he should sit with Siddhâsana, and having performed bandha and Kumbhaka, should begin with 10 Prânâyâmas the first day, and go on increasing 5 daily. 9.

With composed mind 80 Kumbhakas should be performed at a time; beginning first with the chandra (the left nostril) and then sûrya (the right nostril). 10.

This has been spoken of by wise men as Aouloma and Viloma. Having practised Sûrya Bhedan, with Bandhas, the wise rust) should practise Ujjâyî and then Sîtkârî Sîtalî, and Bhastrikâ, he may practice others or not. 11-12.

He should practise mudrâs properly, as instructed by his guru. Then sitting with Padmâsana, he should hear anâhata nâda attentively. 13.

He should resign the fruits of all his practice reverently to God, and, on rising on the completion of the practice, a warm bath should be taken. 14.

The bath should bring all the daily duties briefly to an end. At noon also a little rest should be taken at the end of the exercise, and then food should be taken. 15.

Yogîs should always take wholesome food and never anything unwholesome. After dinner he should eat Ilâchî or lavanga. 16.

Some like camphor, and betel leaf. To the Yogîs, practising Prânâyâma, betel leaf without powders, i, e., lime, nuts and kâtha, is beneficial. 17.

After taking food he should read books treating of salvation, or hear Purânas and repeat the name of God. 18. In the evening the exercise should be begun after finishing sandyhâ, as before, beginning the practice 3 ghatikâ or one hour before the sun sets. 19.

Evening sandhyâ should always be performed after practice, and Hatha Yoga should be practised at midnight. 20.

Viparîta Karni is to be practised in the evening and at midnight, and not just after eating, as it does no good at this time. 21.

51.) atha ujjāyī

mukhaṃ saṃyamya nāḍībhyāmākṛṣhya pava-
naṃ śanaiḥ I yathā laghati kaṇṭhāttu hṛday-
āvadhi sa-svanam

Ujjâyî.

*Having closed the opening of the Nâdî (Larynx), the
air should be drawn in such a way that it goes touching
from the throat to the chest, and making noise while
passing.*

52.) pūrvavatkumbhayetprāṇaṃ rechay-
ediḍayā tathā I śleṣhma-doṣha-haraṃ kaṇṭhe
dehānala-vivardhanam

*It should be restrained, as before, and then let out
through Idâ (the left nostril). This removes ślesmâ (phle-
gm) in the throat and increases the appetite.*

53.) nāḍī-jalodarādhātu-ghata-doṣha-vināśa-
nam I ghachchatā tiṣhṭhatā kāryamujjāyyāk-
hyaṃ tu kumbhakam

*It destroys the defects of the nâdîs, dropsy and disorders
of Dhâtu (humours). Ujjâyî should be performed in all
conditions of life, even while walking or sitting.*

54.) atha sītkārī
sītkāṃ kuryāttathā vaktre ghrāṇenaiva vijṛm-
bhikām | evamabhyāsa-yoghena kāma-devo
dvitīyakaḥ

Sîtkârî.

*Sîtkârî is performed by drawing in the air through the
mouth, keeping the tongue between the lips. The air thus
drawn in should not be expelled through the mouth. By
practising in this way, one becomes next to the God of
Love in beauty.*

55.) yoghinī chakra-sammānyaḥ sṛṣhṭi-
saṃhāra-kārakaḥ | na kṣhudhā na tṛṣhā
nidrā naivālasyaṃ prajāyate

*He is regarded adorable by the Yoginîs and becomes the
destroyer of the cycle of creation, He is not afflicted with
hunger, thirst, sleep or lassitude.*

56.) bhavetsattvaṃ cha dehasya sarvopadra-
va-varjitaḥ | anena vidhinā satyaṃ yoghīnd-
ro bhūmi-maṇḍale

*The Satwa of his body becomes free from all the distur-
bances. In truth, he becomes the lord of the Yogîs in this
world.*

57.) atha śītalī

jihvayā vāyumākṛṣhya pūrvavatkumbha-sād-

hanam ǀ śanakairghrāṇa-randhrābhyāṃ

rechayetpavanaṃ sudhīḥ

Śîtalî.

As in the above (Sîtkári), the tongue to be protruded a little out of the lips, when the air is drawn in. It is kept confined, as before, and then expelled slowly through the nostrils.

58.) ghulma-plīhādikānroghānjvaraṃ pittaṃ

kṣhudhāṃ tṛṣhām ǀ viṣhāṇi śītalī nāma kum-

bhikeyaṃ nihanti hi

This Śîtalî kumbhikâ cures colic, (enlarged) spleen, fever, disorders of bile, hunger, thirst, and counteracts poisons.

59.) atha bhastrikā

ūrvorupari saṃsthāpya śubhe pāda-tale

ubhe ǀ padmāsanaṃ bhavedetatsarva-pā-

pa-praṇāśanam

The Bhastrikâ.

The Padma Âsana consists in crossing the feet and

placing them on both the thighs; it is the destroyer of all sins.

60.) samyakpadmāsanaṃ baddhvā sama-ghrīvodaraḥ sudhīḥ ǀ mukhaṃ saṃya-mya yatnena prāṇaṃ ghrāṇena rechayet

Binding the Padma-Âsana and keeping the body straight, closing the mouth carefully, let the air be expelled through the nose.

61.) yathā laghati hṛt-kaṇṭhe kapālāvad-hi sa-svanam ǀ veghena pūrayechchāpi hṛt-padmāvadhi mārutam

It should be filled up to the lotus of the heart, by drawing it in with force, making noise and touching the throat, the chest and the head.

62.) punarvirechayettadvatpūrayechcha punaḥ punaḥ ǀ yathaiva lohakāreṇa bhastrā veghena chālyate

It should he expelled again and filled again and again as before, just as a pair of bellows of the blacksmith is worked.

**63.) tathaiva sva-śarīra-sthaṃ chālayetpava-
naṃ dhiyā | yadā śramo bhaveddehe tadā
sūryeṇa pūrayet**

*In the same way, the air of the body should be moved
intelligently, filling it through Sûrya when fatigue is
experienced.*

**64.) yathodaraṃ bhavetpūrṇamanilena tathā
laghu | dhārayennāsikāṃ madhyā-tar-
janībhyāṃ vinā dṛḍham**

*The air should be drawn in through the right nostril by
pressing the thumb against the left side of the nose, so
as to close the left nostril; and when filled to the full, it
should be closed with the fourth finger (the one next to
the little finger) and kept confined.*

**65.) vidhivatkumbhakaṃ kṛtvā rechayediḍay-
ānilam | vāta-pitta-śleṣhma-haraṃ śarīrāgh-
ni-vivardhanam**

*Having confined it properly, it should be expelled
through the Idâ (left nostril). This destroys Vâta, pitta
(bile) and phlegm and increases the digestive power (the
gastric fire).*

**66.) kuṇḍalī bodhakam kṣhipram pavanam
sukhadam hitam | brahma-nāḍī-mukhe
samstha-kaphādy-arghala-nāśanam**

*It quickly awakens the Kundalinî, purifies the system,
gives pleasure, and is beneficial. It destroys phlegm
and the impurities accumulated at the entrance of the
Brahma Nâdî.*

**67.) samyaghghātra-samudbhūta-ghrant-
hi-traya-vibhedakam | viśeṣheṇaiva kartavy-
am bhastrākhyam kumbhakam tvidam**

*This Bhastrikâ should be performed plentifully, for it
breaks the three knots: Brahma granthi (in the chest),
Visnu granthi (in the throat), and Rudra granthi
(between the eyebrows) of the body.*

**68.) atha bhrāmarī
veghādghoṣham pūrakam bhṛnggha-nādam
bhṛngghī-nādam rechakam manda-mandam |
yoghīndrāṇamevamabhyāsa-yoghāch chitte
jātā kāchidānanda-līlā**

The Bhrâmari.

By filling the air with force, making noise like Bhringi

*(wasp), and expelling it slowly, making noise in the
same way; this practice causes a sort of ecstacy in the
minds of Yogîndras.*

69.) atha mūrchchā
**pūrakānte ghāḍhataraṃ baddhvā jālandha-
raṃ śanaiḥ | rechayenmūrchchākhyeyaṃ
mano-mūrchchā sukha-pradā**

The Mûrchhâ.

*Closing the passages with Jâlandhar Bandha firmly at
the end of Pûraka, and expelling the air slowly, is called
Mûrchhâ, from its causing the mind to swoon and
giving comfort.*

70.) atha plāvinī
**antaḥ pravartitodāra-mārutāpūritodaraḥ |
payasyaghādhe|api sukhātplavate padma-pa-
travat**

The Plâvinî.

*When the belly is filled with air and the inside of the
body is filled to its utmost with air, the body floats on
the deepest water, like the leaf of a lotus.*

**71.) prāṇāyāmastridhā prokto recha-pūra-
ka-kumbhakaiḥ I sahitaḥ kevalaścheti kum-
bhako dvividho mataḥ**

*Considering Pûraka (Filling), Rechaka (expelling) and
Kumbhaka (confining), Prânâyâma is of three kinds,
but considering it accompanied by Pûraka and Rechaka,
and without these, it is of two kinds only, i.e., Sahita
(with) and Kevala (alone).*

**72.) yāvatkevala-siddhiḥ syātsahitaṃ tāvada-
bhyaset I rechakaṃ pūrakaṃ muktvā suk-
haṃ yadvāyu-dhāraṇam**

*Exercise in Sahita should be continued till success in
Kevala is gained. This latter is simply confining the air
with ease, without Rechaka and Pûraka.*

**73.) prāṇāyāmo|ayamityuktaḥ sa vai keva-
la-kumbhakaḥ I kumbhake kevale siddhe
recha-pūraka-varjite**

*In the practice of Kevala Prânâyâma when it can be
performed successfully without Rechaka and Pûraka,
then it is called Kevala Kumbhaka.*

**74.) na tasya durlabhaṃ kiṃchittriṣhu lo-
keṣhu vidyate I śaktaḥ kevala-kumbhena
yatheṣhṭaṃ vāyu-dhāraṇāt**

*There is nothing in the three worlds which may be
difficult to obtain for him who is able to keep the air
confined according to pleasure, by means of Kevala
Kumbhaka.*

**75.) rāja-yogha-padaṃ chāpi labhate nātra
saṃśayaḥ I kumbhakātkuṇḍalī-bodhaḥ
kuṇḍalī-bodhato bhavet I anarghalā suṣ-
humṇā cha haṭha-siddhiścha jāyate**

*He obtains the position of Râja Yoga undoubtedly. Kun-
dalinî awakens by Kumbhaka, and by its awakening,
Susumnâ becomes free from impurities.*

**76.) haṭhaṃ vinā rājayogho rāja-yoghaṃ vinā
haṭhaḥ I na sidhyati tato yughmamāniṣhpat-
teḥ samabhyaset**

*No success in Râja Yoga without Hatha Yoga, and no
success in Hatha Yoga without Râja Yoga. One should,
therefore, practise both of these well, till complete success
is gained.*

77.) kumbhaka-prāṇa-rodhānte kuryāchchit-tam nirāśrayam | evamabhyāsa-yoghena rāja-yogha-padaṃ vrajet

On the completion of Kumbhaka, the mind should be given rest. By practising in this way one is raised to the position of (succeeds in getting) Râja Yoga.

78.) vapuḥ kṛśatvaṃ vadane prasannatā nā-da-sphuṭatvaṃ nayane sunirmale | aroghatā bindu-jayo|aghni-dīpanaṃ nāḍī-viśuddhir-haṭha-siddhi-lakṣhaṇam

Indications of success in the practice of Hatha Yoga.

When the body becomes lean, the face glows with de-light, Anâhatanâda manifests, and eyes are clear, body is healthy, bindu under control, and appetite increases, then one should know that the Nâdîs are purified and success in Hatha Yoga is approaching.

iti haṭha-pradīpikāyāṃ dvitīyopadeśaḥ

End of Chapter II.

Chapter 3

MUDRAS

Trtīyopadeśah

**1.) sa-śaila-vana-dhātrīṇāṃ yathād-
hāro|ahi-nāyakaḥ | sarveṣhāṃ yogha-tan-
trāṇāṃ tathādhāro hi kuṇḍalī**

*As the chief of the snakes is the support of the earth with
all the mountains and forests on it, so all the Tantras
(Yoga practices) rest on the Kundalinî. (The Vertebral
column.)*

**2.) suptā ghuru-prasādena yadā jāgharti
kuṇḍalī | tadā sarvāṇi padmāni bhidyante
ghranthayo|api cha**

*When the sleeping Kundalinî awakens by favour of a
guru, then all the lotuses (in the six chakras or centres)
and all the knots are pierced through.*

**3.) prāṇasya śūnya-padavī tadā rājapathāy-
ate | tadā chittaṃ nirālambaṃ tadā kālasya
vañchanam**

*Susumnâ (Sûnya Padavî) becomes a main road for the
passage of Prâna, and the mind then becomes free from*

all connections (with its objects of enjoyments) and
Death is then evaded.

4.) suṣhumṇā śūnya-padavī brahma-randhraḥ mahāpathaḥ I śmaśānaṃ śāmbhavī mad-hya-mārghaśchetyeka-vāchakāḥ

Susumnâ, Sunya Padavî, Brahma Randhra, Mahâ Patha, Śmaśâna, Śambhavî, Madhya Mârga, are names of one and the same thing.

5.) tasmātsarva-prayatnena prabodhayi-tumīśvarīm I brahma-dvāra-mukhe suptāṃ mudrābhyāsaṃsamācharet

In order, therefore, to awaken this goddess, who is sleeping at the entrance of Brahma Dwâra (the great door), mudrâs should be practised well.

6.) mahāmudrā mahābandho mahāvedhaścha khecharī I uḍḍīyānaṃ mūlabandhaścha bandho jālandharābhidhaḥ

The mudrâs.

Mahâ Mudrâ, Mahâ Bandha, Mahâ Vedha, Khecharî, Uddiyâna Bandha, Mûla Bandha, Jâlandhara Bandha.

7.) karaṇī viparītākhyā vajrolī śakti-chālanam I idaṃ hi mudrā-daśakaṃ jarā-maraṇa-nāśa-nam

Viparîta Karanî, Vajroli, and Śakti Châlana. These are the ten Mudrâs which annihilate old age and death.

8.) ādināthoditaṃ divyamaṣhṭaiśva-rya-pradāyakam I vallabhaṃ sarva-sidd-hānāṃ durlabhaṃ marutāmapi

They have been explained by Âdi Nâtha (Śiva) and give eight kinds of divine wealth. They are loved by all the Siddhas and are hard to attain even by the Marutas.

Note.—The eight Aiśwaryas are: Animâ (becoming small, like an atom), Mahimâ (becoming great, like âkâs, by drawing in atoms of Prakriti), Garimâ (light things, like cotton becoming very heavy like mountains.)

Prâpti (coming within easy reach of everything; as touching the moon with the little finger, while standing on the earth.)

Prâkâmya (non-resistance to the desires, as entering the earth like water.)

Îsatâ (mastery over matter and objects made of it.)

Vaśitwa (controlling the animate and inanimate objects.)

9.) ghopanīyaṃ prayatnena yathā ratna-ka-raṇḍakam I kasyachinnaiva vaktavyaṃ kula-strī-surataṃ yathā

These Mudrâs should be kept secret by every means, as one keeps one's box of jewellery, and should, on no account be told to any one, just as husband and wife keep their dealings secret.

10.) atha mahā-mudrā
pāda-mūlena vāmena yoniṃ sampīḍya dakṣhiṇāṃ I prasāritaṃ padaṃ kṛtvā karābhyāṃ dhārayeddṛḍham

The mahâ mudrâ.

Pressing the Yoni (perineum) with the heel of the left foot, and stretching forth the right foot, its toe should be grasped by the thumb and first finger.

11+12.) kaṇṭhe bandhaṃ samāropya dhāray-edvāyumūrdhvataḥ I yathā daṇḍa-hataḥ sarpo daṇḍākāraḥ prajāyate

ṛjvībhūtā tathā śaktiḥ kuṇḍalī sahasā bhavet
I tadā sā maraṇāvasthā jāyate dviputāśrayā

*By stopping the throat (by Jâlandhara Bandha) the air
is drawn in from the outside and carried down. Just as a
snake struck with a stick becomes straight like a stick, in
the same way, śakti (susumnâ) becomes straight at once.
Then the Kundalinî, becoming as it were dead, and,*

*leaving both the Idâ and the Pingalâ, enters the su-
sumnâ (the middle passage). 11-12.*

**13.) tataḥ śanaiḥ śanaireva rechayennaiva ve-
ghataḥ I mahā-mudrāṃ cha tenaiva vadanti
vibudhottamāḥ**

*It should be expelled then, slowly only and not violently.
For this very reason, the best of the wise men call it the
Mahâ Mudrâ. This Mahâ Mudrâ has been propounded
by great masters.*

**14.) iyaṃ khalu mahāmudrā mahā-siddhaiḥ
pradarśitā I mahā-kleśādayo doṣhāḥ kṣhīy-
ante maraṇādayaḥ I mahā-mudrāṃ cha
tenaiva vadanti vibudhottamāḥ**

*Great evils and pains, like death, are destroyed by it,
and for this reason wise men call it the Mahâ Mudrâ.*

15.) chandrāngghe tu samabhyasya sūryāngghe punarabhyaset | yāvat-tulyā bhavetsangkhyā tato mudrāṃ visarjayet

Having practised with the left nostril, it should be practised with the right one; and, when the number on both sides becomes equal, then the mudrâ should be discontinued.

16.) na hi pathyamapathyaṃ vā rasāḥ sar-ve|api nīrasāḥ | api bhuktaṃ viṣhaṃ ghoraṃ pīyūṣhamapi jīryati

There is nothing wholesome or injurious; for the practice of this mudrâ destroys the injurious effects of all the rasas (chemicals). Even the deadliest of poisons, if taken, acts like nectar.

17.) kṣhaya-kuṣhṭha-ghudāvarta-ghulmājīrṇa-puroghamāḥ | tasya doṣhāḥ kṣhayaṃ yānti mahāmudrāṃ tu yo|abhyaset

Consumption, leprosy, prolapsus anii, colic, and the diseases due to indigestion, all these irregularities are removed by the practice of this Mahâ Mudrâ.

18.) kathiteyaṃ mahāmudrā mahā-siddhi-karā

nṝṇām | ghopanīyā prayatnena na deyā yasya kasyachit

This Mahâ Mudrâ has been described as the giver of great success (Siddhi) to men. It should be kept secret by every effort, and not revealed to any and everyone.

**19.) atha mahā-bandhaḥ
pārṣhṇiṃ vāmasya pādasya yoni-sthāne niyo-
jayet | vāmorūpari saṃsthāpya dakṣhiṇam
charaṇaṃ tathā**

The Mahâ Bandha.

Press the left heel to the perineum and place the right foot on the left thigh.

**20.) pūrayitvā tato vāyuṃ hṛdaye chubukaṃ
dṛḍham | niṣhpīḍyaṃ vāyumākuñchya ma-
no-madhye niyojayet**

Fill in the air, keeping the chin firm against the chest, and, having pressed the air, the mind should he fixed on the middle of the eyebrows or in the susumnâ (the spine).

**21.) dhārayitvā yathā-śakti rechayedani-
lam śanaiḥ I savyāngghe tu samabhyasya
dakṣhāngghe punarabhyaset**

*Having kept it confined so long as possible, it should
be expelled slowly. Having practised on the left side, it
should be practised on the right side.*

**22.) matamatra tu keṣhāṃchitkaṇṭha-band-
ham vivarjayet I rāja-danta-stha-jihvāyā
bandhaḥ śasto bhavediti**

*Some are of opinion that the closing of throat is not ne-
cessary here, for keeping the tongue pressed against the
roots of the upper teeth makes a good bandha (stop).*

**23.) ayaṃ tu sarva-nāḍīnāmūrdhvaṃ gha-
ti-nirodhakaḥ I ayaṃ khalu mahā-bandho
mahā-siddhi-pradāyakaḥ**

*This stops the upward motion of all the Nâdîs. Verily this
Mahâ Bandha is the giver of great Siddhis.*

**24.) kāla-pāśa-mahā-bandha-vimochana-
vichakṣhaṇaḥ I triveṇī-sangghamaṃ dhatte
kedāraṃ prāpayenmanaḥ**

This Mahâ Bandha is the most skilful means for cutting away the snares of death. It brings about the conjunction of the Trivenî (Idâ, Pingalâ and Susumnâ) and carries the mind to Kedâr (the space between the eyebrows, which is the seat of Śiva).

25.) rūpa-lāvaṇya-sampannā yathā strī puruṣhaṃ vinā | mahā-mudrā-mahā-band-hau niṣhphalau vedha-varjitau

As beauty and loveliness, do not avail a woman without husband, so the Mahâ Mudrâ and the Mahâ-Bandha are useless without the Mahâ Vedha.

26.) atha mahā-vedhaḥ mahā-bandha-sthito yoghī kṛtvā pūrakame-ka-dhīḥ | vāyūnāṃ ghatimāvṛtya nibhṛtaṃ kaṇṭha-mudrayā

The Mahâ Vedha.

Sitting with Mahâ Bandha, the Yogî should fill in the air and keep his mind collected. The movements of the Vâyus (Prâna and Apâna) should be stopped by closing the throat.)

**27.) sama-hasta-yugho bhūmau sphichau
sanāḍayechchanaiḥ | puṭa-dvayamatikramya
vāyuḥ sphurati madhyaghaḥ**

*Resting both the hands equally on the ground, he should
raise himself a little and strike his buttocks against the
ground gently. The air, leaving both the passages (Idâ
and Pingalâ), starts into the middle one.*

**28.) soma-sūryāghni-sambandho jāyate
chāmṛtāya vai | mṛtāvasthā samutpannā tato
vāyuṃ virechayet**

*The union of the Idâ and the Pingalâ is effected, in order
to bring about immortality. When the air becomes as it
were dead (by leaving its course through the Idâ and the
Pingalâ) (i.e., when it has been kept confined), then it
should be expelled.*

**29.) mahā-vedho|ayamabhyāsānmahā-sidd-
hi-pradāyakaḥ | valī-palita-vepa-ghnaḥ sevya-
te sādhakottamaiḥ**

*The practice of this Mahâ Vedha, the giver of great Sidd-
his, destroys old age, grey hair, and shaking of the body,
and therefore it is practised by the best masters.*

30.) etattrayaṃ mahā-ghuhyaṃ jarā-mṛtyu-vināśanam | vahni-vṛddhi-karaṃ chaiva hyaṇimādi-ghuṇa-pradam

These THREE are the great secrets. They are the destroyers of old age and death, increase the appetite, confer the accomplishments of Anima, etc.

31.) aṣhṭadhā kriyate chaiva yāme yāme dine dine | puṇya-saṃbhāra-sandhāya pāpaugha-bhiduraṃ sadā | samyak-śikṣhāvatāmevaṃ svalpaṃ prathama-sādhanam

They should, be practised in 8 ways, daily and hourly. They increase collection of good actions and lessen the evil ones. People, instructed well, should begin their practice, little by little, first.

**32.) atha khecharī
kapāla-kuhare jihvā praviṣhṭā viparītaghā | bhruvorantarghatā dṛṣhṭirmudrā bhavati khecharī**

The Khechari.

The Khechari Mudrâ is accomplished by thrusting the tongue into the gullet, by turning it over itself, and keeping the eyesight in the middle of the eyebrows.

**33.) chedana-chālana-dohaiḥ kalāṃ kra-
meṇātha vardhayettāvat | sā yāvad-
bhrū-madhyaṃ spṛśati tadā khecharī-siddhiḥ**

*To accomplish this, the tongue is lengthened by cutting
the frœnum linguœ, moving, and pulling it. When it can
touch the space between the eyebrows, then Khechari
can be accomplished.*

**34.) snuhī-patra-nibhaṃ śastraṃ sutīkṣhṇaṃ
snighdha-nirmalam | samādāya tatastena
roma-mātraṃ samuchchinet**

*Taking a sharp, smooth, and clean instrument, of the
shape of a cactus leaf, the frœnum of the tongue should
be cut a little (as much as a hair's thickness), at a time.*

**35.) tataḥ saindhava-pathyābhyāṃ
chūrṇitābhyāṃ pragharṣhayet | punaḥ sap-
ta-dine prāpte roma-mātraṃ samuchchinet**

*Then rock salt and yellow myrobalan (both powdered)
should be rubbed in. On the 7th day, it should again be
cut a hair's breadth.*

**36.) evaṃ krameṇa ṣhaṇ-māsaṃ nityaṃ yuk-
taḥ samācharet | ṣhaṇmāsādrasanā-mūla-
śirā-bandhaḥ praṇaśyati**

*One should go on doing thus, regularly for six months.
At the end of six months, the frœnum of the tongue will
be completely cut.*

37.) kalāṃ parāngmukhīṃ kṛtvā tripathe pariyojayet | sā bhavetkhecharī mudrā vyo-ma-chakraṃ taduchyate

*Turning the tongue upwards, it is fixed on the three
ways (œsophagus, windpipe and palate.) Thus it makes
the Khechari Mudrâ, and is called the Vyoma Chakra.*

38.) rasanāmūrdhvaghāṃ kṛtvā kṣhaṇārd-hamapi tiṣhṭhati | viṣhairvimuchyate yoghī vyādhi-mṛtyu-jarādibhiḥ

*The Yogî who sits for a minute turning his tongue
upwards, is saved from poisons, diseases, death, old age,
etc.*

39.) na rogho maraṇaṃ tandrā na nidrā na kṣ-hudhā tṛṣhā | na cha mūrchchā bhavettasya yo mudrāṃ vetti khecharīm

*He who knows the Khechari Mudrâ is not afflicted with
disease, death, sloth, sleep, hunger, thirst, and swooning.*

40.) pīḍyate na sa rogheṇa lipyate na cha karmaṇā | bādhyate na sa kālena yo mudrāṃ vetti khecharīm

He who knows the Khechari Mudrâ, is not troubled by diseases, is not stained with karmas, and is not snared by time.

41.) chittaṃ charati khe yasmājjihvā charati khe ghaṭā | tenaiṣhā khecharī nāma mudrā siddhairnirūpitā

The Siddhas have devised this Khechari Mudrâ from the fact that the mind and the tongue reach âkâśa by its practice.

42.) khecharyā mudritaṃ yena vivaraṃ lam-bikordhvataḥ | na tasya kṣharate binduḥ kāminyāḥ śleṣhitasya cha

If the hole behind the palate be stopped with Khechari by turning the tongue upwards, then bindu cannot leave its place even if a woman were embraced.

43.) chalito|api yadā binduḥ samprāpto yo-ni-maṇḍalam | vrajatyūrdhvaṃ hṛtaḥ śaktyā nibaddho yoni-mudrayā

Even when there is movement of the bindu and it enters the genitals, it is seized by closing the perineum and is taken upward.

44.) ūrdhva-jihvaḥ sthiro bhūtvā somapānaṃ karoti yaḥ I māsārdhena na sandeho mṛtyuṃ jayati yoghavit

If the Yogî drinks Somarasa (juice) by sitting with the tongue turned backwards and mind concentrated, there is no doubt he conquers death within 15 days.

45.) nityaṃ soma-kalā-pūrṇam śarīraṃ yasya yoghinaḥ I takṣhakeṇāpi daṣhṭasya viṣhaṃ tasya na sarpati

The yogi's body is forever full of the moon's nectar. Even if he is bitten by the king of snakes (Takshaka), he is not poisoned

46.) indhanāni yathā vahnistaila-varti cha dī-pakaḥ I tathā soma-kalā-pūrṇam dehī dehaṃ na muñchati

Just as fuel kindles fire and oil a lamp, so the indweller of the body does not vacate while the body is full of the moon's nectar

**47.) ghomāṃsaṃ bhakṣhayennityaṃ pibe-
damara-vāruṇīm I kulīnaṃ tamahaṃ manye
chetare kula-ghātakāḥ**

*By constant swallowing of the tongue he can drink
amaravaruni. I consider him of high lineage (heritage).
Others destroy the heritage.*

**48.) gho-śabdenoditā jihvā tatpraveśo hi
tāluni I gho-māṃsa-bhakṣhaṇaṃ tattu
mahā-pātaka-nāśanam**

*The word 'go' means tongue (and also means cow).
When it enters into the upper palate, it is 'eating the
flesh of the cow.' It (khechari) destroys the great sins.*

**49.) jihvā-praveśa-sambhūta-vahninotpāditaḥ
khalu I chandrātsravati yaḥ sāraḥ sā syāda-
mara-vāruṇī**

*When the tongue enters the cavity, indeed heat is produ-
ced and the man's nectar flows.*

**50.) chumbantī yadi lambikāghramaniśaṃ
jihvā-rasa-syandinī sa-kṣhārā kaṭukām-
la-dughdha-sadṛśī madhvājya-tulyā tathā
I vyādhīnāṃ haraṇaṃ jarānta-karaṇam**

**śastrāghamodīraṇaṃ tasya syādamaratva-
maṣhṭa-ghuṇitaṃ siddhāngghanākarṣhaṇam**

*When the tongue constantly presses the cavity, the
moon's nectar (flows and) has a saline, pungent and
acidic flavor. It is like (the consistency of) milk, ghee,
honey. Fatal diseases, old age and weapons are warded
off. From that, immortality and the eight siddhis or
perfections manifest.*

**51.) ūrdvhāsyo rasanāṃ niyamya vivare śak-
tiṃ parāṃ chintayan | utkallola-kalā-jalaṃ
cha vimalaṃ dhārāmayaṃ yaḥ piben nirvyād-
hiḥ sa mṛṇāla-komala-vapuryoghī chiraṃ
jīvati**

*Fluid drips into the sixteen petalled lotus (vishuddhi
chakra) when the tongue is inserted into the upper
throat cavity; the paramshakti (kundalini) is released
and one becomes concentrated in that (experience which
ensues). The yogi who drinks the pure stream of nectar
is freed from disease, has longevity, and has a body as
soft and as beautiful as a lotus stem.*

**52.) yatprāleyaṃ prahita-suṣhiraṃ
meru-mūrdhāntara-sthaṃ tasmiṃstattvaṃ
pravadati sudhīstan-mukhaṃ nimnaghānām**

I chandrātsāraḥ sravati vapuṣhastena mṛty-
urnarāṇāṃ tadbadhnīyātsukaraṇamadho
nānyathā kāya-siddhiḥ

*The nectar is secreted from the topmost part of the
Meru (Sushumna), the fountainhead of the nadis. He
who has pure intellect can know the Truth therein. The
nectar, which is the essence of the body, flows out from
the moon and hence death ensues. Therefore khechari
mudra should be practiced, otherwise perfection of the
body cannot be attained.*

**53.) suṣhiraṃ jñāna-janakaṃ pañcha-sro-
taḥ-samanvitam I tiṣhṭhate khecharī mudrā
tasminśūnye nirañjane**

*Five nadis convene in this cavity and it is the source of
knowledge. Khechari should be established in that void,
untainted (by ignorance).*

**54.) ekaṃ sṛṣhṭimayaṃ bījamekā mudrā cha
khecharī I eko devo nirālamba ekāvasthā
manonmanī**

*There is only one seed of creation and one mudra –
khechari; one deva independent of everything and one
state – manonmani.*

**55.) atha uḍḍīyāna-bandhaḥ
baddho yena suṣhumṇāyāṃ prāṇastūḍḍīyate
yataḥ | tasmāduḍḍīyanākhyo|ayaṃ yog-
hibhiḥ samudāhṛtaḥ**

The Uddiyâna bandha.

*Uddiyana bandha is so-called by the yogis because
through its practice the prana (is concentrated at one
point and) rises through sushumna.*

**56.) uḍḍīnaṃ kurute yasmādaviśrāntaṃ
mahā-khaghaḥ | uḍḍīyānaṃ tadeva syāttava
bandho|abhidhīyate**

*The bandha described is called the rising or flying band-
ha, because through its practice, the great bird (shakti)
flies upward with ease.*

**57.) udare paśchimaṃ tānaṃ nābherūrdh-
vaṃ cha kārayet | uḍḍīyāno hyasau bandho
mṛtyu-mātanggha-kesarī**

*Pulling the abdomen back in and making the navel rise
is uddiyana bandha. It is the lion which conquers the
elephant, death.*

58.) uḍḍīyānaṃ tu sahajaṃ ghuruṇā kathitaṃ sadā | abhyasetsatataṃ yastu vṛddho|api taruṇāyate

Uddiyana is easy when practiced as told by the guru. Even an old person can become young when it is done regularly.

59.) nābherūrdhvamadhaśchāpi tānaṃ kuryātprayatnataḥ | ṣhaṇmāsamabhyasen-mṛtyuṃ jayatyeva na saṃśayaḥ

The region above and below the navel should be drawn backward with effort. There is no doubt that after six months of practice, death is conquered.

60.) sarveṣhāmeva bandhānāṃ uttamo hyuḍḍīyānakaḥ | uḍḍiyāne dṛḍhe bandhe muktiḥ svābhāvikī bhavet

Of all the bandhas, uddiyana is the best. Once it is mastered, mukti or liberation occurs spontaneously.

**61.) atha mūla-bandhaḥ
pārṣhṇi-bhāghena sampīḍya yonimākuñchay-edghudam | apānamūrdhvamākṛṣhya mūla-bandho|abhidhīyate**

The Moola bhanda.

Pressing the perineum/vagina with the heel and contracting the rectum so that the apana vayu moves upward is moola bandha.

62.) adho-ghatimapānaṃ vā ūrdhvaghaṃ kurute balāt I ākuñchanena taṃ prā-hurmūla-bandhaṃ hi yoghinaḥ

By contracting the perineum the downward moving apana vayu is forced to go upward. Yogis call this moola bandha.

63.) ghudaṃ pārṣhṇyā tu sampīḍya vāy-umākuñchayedbalāt I vāraṃ vāraṃ yathā chordhvaṃ samāyāti samīraṇaḥ

Press the heel firmly against the rectum and contract forcefully and repeatedly, so that the vital energy rises.

64.) prāṇāpānau nāda-bindū mūla-bandhena chaikatām I ghatvā yoghasya saṃsiddhiṃ yachchato nātra saṃśayaḥ

There is no doubt that by practicing moola bandha, prana/apana and nada/bindu are united, and total perfection attained.

65.) apāna-prāṇayoraikyaṃ kṣhayo mūtra-purīṣhayoḥ I yuvā bhavati vṛddho|api satataṃ mūla-bandhanāt

With constant practice of moola bandha, prana and apana unite, urine and stool are decreased and even an old person becomes young.

66.) apāna ūrdhvaghe jāte prayāte vah-ni-maṇḍalam I tadānala-śikhā dīrghā jāyate vāyunāhatā

Apana moves up into the region of fire (manipura chakra, the navel center), then the flames of the fire grow, being fanned by apana vayu.

67.) tato yāto vahny-apānau prāṇamuṣhṇa-svarūpakam I tenātyan-ta-pradīptastu jvalano dehajastathā

Then, when apana and the fin meet with prana, which is itself hot, the heat in the body is intensified.

68.) tena kuṇḍalinī suptā santaptā sampra-budhyate I daṇḍāhatā bhujangghīva niśvasya ṛjutāṃ vrajet

Through this, the sleeping kundalini is aroused by the extreme heat and it straightens itself just as a serpent beaten with a stick straightens and hisses.

69.) bilaṃ praviṣṭeva tato brahma-nāḍyaṃ taraṃ vrajet I tasmānnityaṃ mūla-bandhaḥ kartavyo yoghibhiḥ sadā

Just as a snake enters its hole, so kundalini goes into brahma nadi. Therefore the yogi must always perform moola bandha.

70.) atha jalandhara-bandhaḥ kaṇṭhamākuñchya hṛdaye sthāpayechchibu-kaṃ dṛḍham I bandho jālandharākhyoǀayaṃ jarā-mṛtyu-vināśakaḥ

The Jâlandhara Bandha.

Contracting the throat by bringing the chin to the chest is the bandha called jalandhara. It destroys old age and death.

71.) badhnāti hi sirājālamadho-ghāmi nabho-jalam I tato jālandharo bandhaḥ kaṇṭha-duḥkhaugha-nāśanaḥ

That is jalandhara bandha which catches the flow of nectar in the throat. It destroys all throat ailments.

72.) jālandhare kṛte bandhe kaṇṭha-saṃko-cha-lakṣhaṇe I na pīyūṣhaṃ patatyaghnau na cha vāyuḥ prakupyati

Having done jalandhara bandha by contracting the throat, the nectar does not fall into the gastric fire and the prana is not agitated.

73.) kaṇṭha-saṃkochanenaiva dve nāḍyau stambhayeddṛḍham I madhya-chakramidaṃ jñeyaṃ ṣhoḍaśādhāra-bandhanam

The two Nâdîs should be stopped firmly by contracting the throat. This is called the middle circuit or centre (Madhya Chakra), and it stops the 16 âdhâras (i.e., vital parts).

Note.

The sixteen vital parts mentioned by renowned Yogîs are the (1) thumbs, (2) ankles, (3) knees, (4) thighs, (5) the prepuce, (6) organs of generation, (17) the navel, (8) the heart, (9) the neck, (10) the throat, (11) the palate, (12) the nose, (13) the middle of the eyebrows, (14) the forehead, (15) the head and (16) the Brahma randhra.

74.) mūla-sthānaṃ samākuñchya uḍḍiyānaṃ tu kārayet I iḍāṃ cha pingghalāṃ baddhvā vāhayetpaśchime pathi

By drawing up the mûlasthâna (anus,) Uddiyâna Bandha should be performed. The flow of the air should be directed to the Susumnâ, by closing the Idâ, and the Pingalâ. 73.

75.) anenaiva vidhānena prayāti pavano layam I tato na jāyate mṛtyurjarā-roghādikaṃ tathā

The Prâna becomes calm and latent by this means, and thus there is no death, old age, disease, etc.

76.) bandha-trayamidaṃ śreṣhṭhaṃ mahā-siddhaiścha sevitam I sarveṣhāṃ haṭha-tantrāṇāṃ sādhanaṃ yoghino viduḥ

These three Bandhas are the best of all and have been practised by the masters. Of all the means of success in the Hatha Yoga, they are known to the Yogîs as the chief ones.

77.) yatkiṃchitsravate chandrādamṛtaṃ divya-rūpiṇaḥ I tatsarvaṃ ghrasate sūryastena piṇḍo jarāyutaḥ

That nectar which flows from the moon has the quality of endowing enlightenment, but it is completely consumed by the sun, incurring old age.

78.) atha viparīta-karaṇī mudrā
tatrāsti karaṇam divyaṃ sūryasya muk-
ha-vañchanam | ghurūpadeśato jñeyaṃ na tu
śāstrārtha-koṭibhiḥ

The Viparîta Karani.

There is a wonderful means by which the nectar is averted from falling into the opening of the sun. This is obtained by the guru's instructions and not from the hundreds of shastras (treatises).

79.) ūrdhva-nābheradhastālorūrdhvaṃ
bhānuradhaḥ śaśī | karaṇī viparītākhā ghu-
ru-vākyena labhyate

With the navel region above and the palate below, the sun is above and the moon below. It is called vipareeta karani, the reversing process. When given by the guru's instructions it is fruitful.

80.) nityamabhyāsa-yuktasya jaṭharāghni-vi-
vardhanī | āhāro bahulastasya sampādyaḥ
sādhakasya cha

Digestion is strengthened by continual, regular practice and therefore, the practitioner should always have sufficient food.

81.) alpāhāro yadi bhavedaghnirdahati tat-kshaṇāt | adhaḥ-śirāśchordhva-pādaḥ kshaṇaṃ syātprathame dine

If one takes only a little food, the heat produced by the digestion will destroy the system. Therefore, on the first day, one should only stay a moment with the feet up and head down.

82.) kshaṇāchcha kiṃchidadhikamabhya-sechcha dine dine | valitaṃ palitaṃ chaiva shaṇmāsordhvaṃ na dṛśyate | yāma-mātraṃ tu yo nityamabhyasetsa tu kālajit

The practice should be done daily, gradually increasing the duration. After six months of practice, grey hairs and wrinkles become inconspicuous. One who practices it for yama (three hours conquers death.

83.) atha vajrolī svechchayā vartamāno|api yoghoktairniy-amairvinā | vajrolīṃ yo vijānāti sa yoghī siddhi-bhājanam

The Vajroli.

Even anyone living a free lifestyle without the formal rules of yoga, if he practices vajroli well, that yogi becomes a recipient of siddhis (perfections).

84.) tatra vastu-dvayaṃ vakṣhye durlabhaṃ yasya kasyachit | kṣhīraṃ chaikaṃ dvitīyaṃ tu nārī cha vaśa-vartinī

There are two things hard to obtain, one is milk and the second is a woman who can act according to your will.

85.) mehanena śanaiḥ samyaghūrdh-vākuñchanamabhyaset | puruṣho|apyathavā nārī vajrolī-siddhimāpnuyāt

By practicing gradual upward contractions during the emission in intercourse, any man or woman achieves perfection of vajroli.

86.) yatnataḥ śasta-nālena phūtkāraṃ vaj-ra-kandare | śanaiḥ śanaiḥ prakurvīta vāyu-saṃchāra-kāraṇāt

By slowly drawing in air through a prescribed tube inserted into the urethra of the penis, gradually air and prana traverse into the vajra kanda.

**87.) nārī-bhaghe padad-bindumabhyāsenord-
hvamāharet | chalitaṃ cha nijaṃ bindumūrd-
hvamākṛṣhya rakṣhayet**

*The bindu (semen) that is about to fall into the woman's
vagina should be made to move upwards with practice.
And if it falls, the semen and the woman's fluid should
be conserved by drawing it up.*

**88.) evaṃ saṃrakṣhayedbinduṃ jayati
yoghavit | maraṇaṃ bindu-pātena jīvanaṃ
bindu-dhāraṇāt**

*Therefore, the knower of yoga conquers death by pre-
serving the bindu (semen). Release of the bindu means
death; conservation of semen is life.*

**89.) sughandho yoghino dehe jāyate bin-
du-dhāraṇāt | yāvadbinduḥ sthiro dehe
tāvatkāla-bhayaṃ kutaḥ**

*As long as the bindu/semen is steady in the body, then
where is the fear of death? The yogi's body smells plea-
sant by conserving the bindu/semen.*

**90.) chittāyattaṃ nṛṇāṃ śukraṃ śukrāyattaṃ
cha jīvitam | tasmāchchukraṃ manaśchaiva
rakṣhaṇīyaṃ prayatnataḥ**

A man's semen can be controlled by the mind and control of semen is life giving. Therefore, his semen and mind should be controlled and conserved.

91.) ṛtumatyā rajo|apyevaṃ nijaṃ binduṃ ch rakṣhayet I meḍhreṇākarṣhayedūrdhvaṃ samyaghabhyāsa-yogha-vit

The knower of yoga, perfect in the practice, conserves his bindu and the woman's rajas by drawing it up through the generative organ.

92.) atha sahajoliḥ sahajoliśchāmarolirvajrolyā bheda ekataḥ I jale subhasma nikṣhipya daghdha-gho-maya-sambhavam

The Sahajolî.

Sahajoli and amaroli are separate techniques of vajroli. The ashes of burnt cow manure should be mixed with water.

93.) vajrolī-maithunādūrdhvaṃ strī-puṃsoḥ svāngha-lepanam I āsīnayoḥ sukhenaiva mukta-vyāpārayoḥ kṣhaṇāt

After performing vajroli during intercourse, (being in a comfortable position), the man and woman should wipe the ashes on specific parts of their bodies during the leisure time.

94.) sahajoliriyaṃ proktā śraddheyā yog-hibhiḥ sadā I ayaṃ śubhakaro yogho bhog-ha-yukto|api muktidaḥ

It is called sahajoli and the yogis have complete faith in it. This is very beneficial and enables enlightenment through the combination of yoga and bhoga (sensual involvement).

95.) ayaṃ yoghaḥ puṇyavatāṃ dhīrāṇāṃ tatt-va-darśinām I nirmatsarāṇāṃ vai sidhyenna tu matsara-śālinām

Verily this yoga is perfected by virtuous and well-conducted men who have seen the truth and not those who are selfish.

96.) atha amarolī pittolbaṇatvātprathamāmbu-dhārāṃ vihāya niḥsāratayāntyadhārām I niṣhevyate śīta-la-madhya-dhārā kāpālike khaṇḍamate|a-marolī

The Amaroli.

According to the Kapalika sect, amaroli is practiced by drinking the cool midstream of urine. The first part of the urine is left as it contains bile, and the last part is left as it does not contain goodness.

97.) amarīṃ yaḥ pibennityaṃ nasyaṃ kurvandine dine | vajrolīmabhyasetsamyaksāmarolīti kathyate

One who drinks amari, takes it through the nose and practices vajroli, is said to be practicing amaroli.

98.) abhyāsānnihsṛtāṃ chāndrīṃ vibhūtyā saha miśrayet | dhārayeduttamānggheṣhu divya-dṛṣhṭiḥ prajāyate

The practitioner should mix the semen with the ashes of burnt cow manure and wipe it on the upper parts of the body, it bestows divya drishti (clairvoyance or divine sight).

99.) puṃso binduṃ samākuñchya samyaghabhyāsa-pāṭavāt | yadi nārī rajo rakṣhedvajrolyā sāpi yoghinī

If a woman practices vajroli and saves her rajas and the man's bindu by thorough contraction, she is a yogini.

100.) tasyāḥ kiṃchidrajo nāśaṃ na ghach-chati na saṃśayaḥ | tasyāḥ śarīre nādaścha bindutāmeva ghachchati

Without doubt, not even a little rajas is wasted through vajroli, the nada and bindu in the body become one.

101.) sa bindustadrajaśchaiva ekībhūya sva-dehaghau | vajroly-abhyāsa-yoghena sar-va-siddhiṃ prayachchataḥ

The bindu and that rajas in one's own body unite through the union by practice of vajroli, thus bestowing all perfections or siddhis.

102.) rakṣhedākuñchanādūrdhvaṃ yā rajaḥ sā hi yoghinī | atītānāghataṃ vetti khecharī cha bhaveddhruvam

She is verily a yogini who conserves her rajas by contracting and raising it. She knows past, present and future and becomes fixed in khechari (i.e. consciousness moves into the higher realm).

**103.) deha-siddhiṃ cha labhate vaj-
roly-abhyāsa-yoghataḥ | ayaṃ puṇya-karo
yogho bhoghe bhukte | api muktidaḥ**

*By the yoga of vajroli practice, perfection of the body
fructifies. This auspicious yoga even brings liberation
alongside with sensual involvement (bhoga).*

**104.) atha śakti-chālanam
kuṭilāngghī kuṇḍalinī bhujangghī śaktirīśvarī
| kuṇḍalyarundhatī chaite śabdāḥ pa-
ryāya-vāchakāḥ**

The Śakti châlana.

*Kutilangi, kundalini, bhujangi, shakti, ishwari, kundali,
arundhati are all synonymous terms.*

**105.) udghāṭayetkapāṭaṃ tu yathā kuṃchi-
kayā haṭhāt | kuṇḍalinyā tathā yoghī
mokṣhadvāraṃ vibhedayet**

*Just as a door is opened with a key, similarly the yogi
opens the door to liberation with kundalini.*

**106.) yena mārgheṇa ghantavyaṃ brahma-st-
hānaṃ nirāmayam | mukhenāchchhādya
tadvāraṃ prasuptā parameśvarī**

The sleeping Parameshwari rests with her mouth closing that door, through which is the path to the knot of brahmasthana, the place beyond suffering.

107.) kandordhve kuṇḍalī śaktiḥ suptā mokṣhāya yoghinām | bandhanāya cha mūḍhānāṃ yastāṃ vetti sa yoghavit

The kundalini shakti sleeps above the kanda. This shakti is the means of liberation to the yogi and bondage for the ignorant.

One who knows this is the knower of yoga.

108.) kuṇḍalī kuṭilākārā sarpavatparikīrtitā | sā śaktiśchālitā yena sa mukto nātra saṃśayaḥ

Kundalini is said to be coiled like a snake. **Without a doubt, one who makes that shakti flow obtains liberation.**

109.) ghanggghā-yamunayormadhye bāla-raṇḍāṃ tapasvinīm | balātkāreṇa ghṛhṇīyāt-tadviṣhṇoḥ paramaṃ padam

Between Ganga and Yamuna is the young widowed,

Balarandam practicing austerity. She should be seized forcibly, then one can reach the supreme state of Vishnu.

110.) iḍā bhaghavatī ghanggha pingghalā yamunā nadī ǀ iḍā-pingghalayormadhye bālaraṇḍā cha kuṇḍalī

Ida is the holy Ganga, pingala the river Yamuna. Between ida and pingala in the middle is this young widow, kundalini.

111.) puchche praghṛhya bhujangghīṃ suptāmudbodhayechcha tām ǀ nidrāṃ vihāya sā śaktirūrdhvamuttiṣhṭhate haṭhāt

By seizing the tail of kundalini serpent, she becomes very excited. Abandoning sleep that shakti is released and rises up.

112.) avasthitā chaiva phaṇāvatī sā prātaścha sāyaṃ praharārdha-mātram ǀ prapūrya sūryātparidhāna-yuktyā praghṛhya nityaṃ parichālanīyā

Shakti Chalana Mudra.

Breathing in through the right nostril (pingala) the

*serpent (shakti) should be seized through kumbhaka
and rotated constantly for an hour and a half, morning
and evening.*

113.) ūrdhvaṃ vitasti-mātraṃ tu vistāraṃ cha-turangghulam I mṛdulaṃ dhavalaṃ proktaṃ veṣhṭitāmbara-lakṣhaṇam

*The kanda, situated above the anus, one hand span
high and four fingers breath wide, is soft and white as if
enveloped in cloth.*

114.) sati vajrāsane pādau karābhyāṃ dhāray-eddṝḍham I ghulpha-deśa-samīpe cha kan-daṃ tatra prapīḍayet

*Firmly seated in vajrasana, holding the ankles, one
should squeeze the kanda close to the anus.*

115.) vajrāsane sthito yoghī chālayitvā cha kuṇḍalīm I kuryādanantaraṃ bhastrāṃ kuṇḍalīmāśu bodhayet

*In the position of vajrasana, the yogi should move the
kundalini. Having done bhastrika pranayama the kun-
dalini is soon aroused.*

**116.) bhānorākuñchanaṃ kuryātkuṇḍalīṃ
chālayettataḥ | mṛtyu-vaktra-ghatasyāpi
tasya mṛtyu-bhayaṃ kutaḥ**

*Contracting the sun in manipura, kundalini should be
moved. Even if such a person should be on the verge of
death, where is the need to fear death?*

**117.) muhūrta-dvaya-paryantaṃ nirbhay-
am chālanādasau | ūrdhvamākṛṣhyate
kiṃchitsuṣhumṇāyāṃ samudghatā**

*By moving the kundalini fearlessly for an hour and a
half, it is drawn into sushumna and rises up a little.*

**118.) tena kuṇḍalinī tasyāḥ suṣhumṇāyā
mukhaṃ dhruvam | jahāti tasmātprāṇo|ayaṃ
suṣhumṇāṃ vrajati svataḥ**

*In this way, it is easy for kundalini to issue from the
opening of sushumna. Thus the prana proceeds through
sushumna of its own accord.*

**119.) tasmātsaṃchālayennityaṃ sukha-suptā-
marundhatīm | tasyāḥ saṃchālanenaiva
yoghī roghaiḥ pramuchyate**

In that way the sleeping kundalini should be regularly moved. By her regular movement, the yogi is freed from disease.

120.) yena saṃchālitā śaktiḥ sa yoghī siddhi-bhājanam | kimatra bahunoktena kālaṃ jayati līlayā

The yogi who moves the shakti regularly, enjoys perfection or siddhi. He easily conquers time and death. What more is there to say?

121.) brahmacharya-ratasyaiva nityaṃ hita-mitāśinaḥ | maṇḍalāddṛśyate siddhiḥ kuṇḍaly-abhyāsa-yoghinaḥ

One who enjoys being brahmacharya and always takes moderate diet and practices arousal of kundalini, achieves perfection in forty days.

122.) kuṇḍalīṃ chālayitvā tu bhastrāṃ kuryādviśeṣhataḥ | evamabhyasyato nityaṃ yamino yama-bhīḥ kutaḥ

Bhastrika pranayama with kumbhaka should specifically be practiced to activate kundalini. From where will the fear of death arise for a self- restrained practitioner who practices daily with regularity?

**123.) dvā-saptati-sahasrāṇāṃ nāḍīnāṃ
mala-śodhane ǀ kutaḥ prakṣhālanopāyaḥ
kuṇḍaly-abhyasanādṛte**

*What other methods are there to cleanse the 72,000
nadis of dirt besides the practice of arousing kundalini?*

**124.) iyaṃ tu madhyamā nāḍī dṛḍhābhyāsena
yoghinām ǀ āsana-prāṇa-saṃyāma-mud-
rābhiḥ saralā bhavet**

*This middle nadi, sushumna, easily becomes establis-
hed, (straight) by the yogi's persistent practice of asana,
pranayama, mudra and concentration.*

**125.) abhyāse tu vinidrāṇāṃ mano dhṛtvā
samādhinā ǀ rudrāṇī vā parā mudrā bhadrāṃ
siddhiṃ prayachchati**

*For those who are alert and the mind one-pointed (dis-
ciplined) in samadhi, rudrani or shambhavi mudra is
the greatest mudra for bestowing perfection.*

**126.) rāja-yoghaṃ vinā pṛthvī rāja-yoghaṃ
vinā niśā ǀ rāja-yoghaṃ vinā mudrā vichitrā-
pi na śobhate**

The earth without raja yoga, night without raja yoga,
even the various mudras without raja yoga are useless,
i.e. not beautiful.

127.) mārutasya vidhiṃ sarvaṃ mano-yuktaṃ samabhyaset I itaratra na kartavyā mano-vṛt-tirmanīṣhiṇā

All the pranayama methods are to be done with a con-
centrated mind. The wise man should not let his mind
be involved in the modifications (vrittis).

128.) iti mudrā daśa proktā ādināthena śam-bhunā I ekaikā tāsu yamināṃ mahā-sidd-hi-pradāyinī

Thus the ten mudras have been told by Adinath,
Shambhu. Each one is the bestower of perfection to the
self-restrained.

129.) upadeśaṃ hi mudrāṇāṃ yo datte sāmpradāyikam I sa eva śrī-ghuruḥ svāmī sākṣhādīśvara eva saḥ

One who instructs mudra in the tradition of guru/disci-
ple is the true guru and form of Ishwara.

**130.) tasya vākya-paro bhūtvā mudrābhyā-
se samāhitaḥ l aṇimādi-ghuṇaiḥ sārdhaṃ
labhate kāla-vañchanam**

*By following explicitly his (guru's) words, and practicing
mudra; one obtains the qualities of anima, etc. and
overcomes death/time*

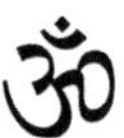

iti haṭha-pradīpikāyāṃ tṛtīyopadeśaḥ

End of chapter III, on the Exposition of the Mudrâs.

Chapter 4
Samadhi
Chaturthopadeśah

**1.) namaḥ śivāya ghurave nāda-bindu-kalāt-
mane I nirañjana-padaṃ yāti nityaṃ tatra
parāyaṇaḥ**

*Salutation to the Gurû, the dispenser of happiness to
all, appearing as Nâda, Vindû and Kalâ. One who is
devoted to Him, obtains the highest bliss.*

**2.) athedānīṃ pravakṣhyāmi samādhikra-
mamuttamam I mṛtyughnaṃ cha sukhopāy-
aṃ brahmānanda-karaṃ param**

*Now I will describe a regular method of attaining to
Samâdhi, which destroys death, is the means for obtai-
ning happiness, and gives the Brahmânanda.*

**3+4.) rāja-yoghaḥ samādhiścha unmanī
cha manonmanī I amaratvaṃ layastattvaṃ
śūnyāśūnyaṃ paraṃ padam**

**amanaskaṃ tathādvaitaṃ nirālambaṃ nirañ-
janam I jīvanmuktiścha sahajā turyā chety-
eka-vāchakāḥ**

*Raja Yogî, Samâdhi, Unmani, Mauonmanî, Amarativa,
Laya, Tatwa, Sûnya, Aśûnya, Parama Pada, Amanas-
ka, Adwaitama, Nirālamba, Nirañjana, Jîwana Mukti,
Sahajâ, Turyâ, are all synonymous.*

5.) salile saindhavaṃ yadvatsāmyaṃ bhajati yoghataḥ | tathātma-manasoraikyaṃ samādhirabhidhīyate

*As salt being dissolved in water becomes one with it, so
when Âtmâ and mind become one, it is called Samâdhi.*

6.) yadā saṃkṣhīyate prāṇo mānasaṃ cha pralīyate | tadā samarasatvaṃ cha samādhirabhidhīyate

*When the Prâna becomes lean (vigourless) and the
mind becomes absorbed, then their becoming equal is
called Samâdhi.*

7.) tat-samaṃ cha dvayoraikyaṃ jīvātma-paramātmanoḥ | pranaṣhṭa-sarva-sangkalpaḥ samādhiḥ so|abhidhīyate

*This equality and oneness of the self and the ultra self,
when all Sankalpas cease to exist, is called Samâdhi.*

8.) rāja-yoghasya māhātmyaṃ ko vā jānāti tattvataḥ ǀ jñānaṃ muktiḥ sthitiḥ siddhirghu-ru-vākyena labhyate

Or, who can know the true greatness of the Raja Yoga. Knowledge, mukti, condition, and Siddhîs can be learnt by instructions from a gurû alone.

9.) durlabho viṣhaya-tyāgho durlabhaṃ tattva-darśanam ǀ durlabhā sahajāvasthā sad-ghuroḥ karuṇāṃ vinā

Indifference to worldly enjoyments is very difficult to obtain, and equally difficult is the knowledge of the Realities to obtain. It is very difficult to get the condition of Samâdhi, without the favour of a true guru.

10.) vividhairāsanaih kubhairvichitraih ka-raṇairapi ǀ prabuddhāyāṃ mahā-śaktau prāṇaḥ śūnye pralīyate

By means of various postures and different Kumbha-kas, when the great power (Kundalî) awakens, then the Prâna becomes absorbed in Sûnya (Samâdhi).

11.) utpanna-śakti-bodhasya tyak-ta-niḥśeṣha-karmaṇaḥ ǀ yoghinaḥ sa-hajāvasthā svayameva prajāyate

The Yogî whose śakti has awakened, and who has reno-
unced all actions, attains to the condition of Samâdhi,
without any effort.

12.) suṣhumṇā-vāhini prāṇe śūnye viśati mānase | tadā sarvāṇi karmāṇi nirmūlayati yoghavit

When the Prâna flows in the Susumnâ, and the mind
has entered śûnya, then the Yogî is free from the effects
of Karmas.

13.) amarāya namastubhyaṃ so|api kālast- vayā jitaḥ | patitaṃ vadane yasya jaghade- tachcharācharam

O Immortal one (that is, the yogi who has attained to
the condition of Samâdhi), I salute thee! Even death
itself, into whose mouth the whole of this movable and
immovable world has fallen, has been conquered by
thee.

14.) chitte samatvamāpanne vāyau vraja- ti madhyame | tadāmarolī vajrolī sahajolī prajāyate

Amarolî, Vajrolî and Sahajolî are accomplished when

the mind becomes calm and Prâna has entered the middle channel.

15.) jñānaṃ kuto manasi sambhavatīha tāvat prāṇo|api jīvati mano mriyate na yāvat | prāṇo mano dvayamidaṃ vilayaṃ nayedyo mokṣhaṃ sa ghachchati naro na kathaṃchi-danyaḥ

How can it he possible to get knowledge, so long as the Prâna is living and the mind has not died? No one else can get moksa, except one who can make one's Prâna and mind latent.

16.) jñātvā suṣhumṇāsad-bhedaṃ kṛtvā vāyuṃ cha madhyagham | sthitvā sadaiva susthāne brahma-randhre nirodhayet

Always living in a good locality and having known the secret of the Susumnâ, which has a middle course, and making the Vâyu move in it., (the Yogî) should restrain the Vâyu in the Brahma randhra.

17.) sūrya-chandramasau dhattaḥ kālaṃ rātrindivātmakam | bhoktrī suṣhumnā kālasya ghuhyametadudāhṛtam

Time, in the form of night and day, is made by the sun and the moon. That, the Susumnâ devours this time (death) even, is a great secret.

18.) dvā-saptati-sahasrāṇi nāḍī-dvārāṇi pañja-re l suṣhumṇā śāmbhavī śaktiḥ śeṣhāstveva nirarthakāḥ

In this body there are 72,000 openings of Nâdis; of these, the Susumnâ, which has the Sâmhhavî Sakti in it, is the only important one, the rest are useless.

19.) vāyuḥ parichito yasmādaghninā saha kuṇḍalīm l bodhayitvā suṣhumṇāyāṃ pra-viśedanirodhataḥ

The Vâyu should be made to enter the Susumnâ without restraint by him who has practised the control of bre-athing and has awakened the Kundali by the (gastric) fire.

20.) suṣhumṇā-vāhini prāṇe siddhyatyeva manonmanī l anyathā tvitarābhyāsāḥ pray-āsāyaiva yoghinām

The Prâna, flowing through the Susumnâ, brings about the condition of manonmanî; other practices are simply futile for the Yogî.

**21.) pavano badhyate yena manastenaiva
badhyate | manaścha badhyate yena pava-
nastena badhyate**

*By whom the breathing has been controlled, by him the
activities of the mind also have been controlled; and,
conversely, by whom the activities of the mind have been
controlled, by him the breathing also has been control-
led.*

**22.) hetu-dvayaṃ tu chittasya vāsanā cha
samīraṇaḥ | tayorvinaṣhṭa ekasmintau dvāva-
pi vinaśyataḥ**

*There are two causes of the activities of the mind: (1)
Vâsanâ (desires) and (2) the respiration (the Prâna).
Of these, the destruction of the one is the destruction of
both.*

**23.) mano yatra vilīyeta pavanastatra līyate |
pavano līyate yatra manastatra vilīyate**

*Breathing is lessened when the mind becomes absorbed,
and the mind becomes absorbed when the Prâna is
restrained.*

24.) dughdhāmbuvatsaṃmilitāvubhau tau tulya-kriyau mānasa-mārutau hi I yato maruttatra manaḥ-pravṛttir yato manastatra marut-pravṛttiḥ

Both the mind and the breath are united together, like milk and water; and both of them are equal in their activities. Mind begins its activities where there is the breath, and the Parana begins its activities where there is the mind.

25.) atraika-nāśādaparasya nāśa eka-pravṛt-terapara-pravṛttiḥ I adhvastayośchend-riya-vargha-vṛttiḥ pradhvastayormokṣha-pa-dasya siddhiḥ

By the suspension of the one, therefore, comes the suspension of the other, and by the operations of the one are brought about the operations of the other. When they are present, the Indriyas (the senses) remain engaged in their proper functions, and when they become latent then there is moksa.

26.) rasasya manasaśchaiva chañchalatvaṃ svabhāvataḥ I raso baddho mano baddhaṃ kiṃ na siddhyati bhūtale

*By nature, Mercury and mind are unsteady: there is
nothing in the world which cannot be accomplished
when these are made steady.*

27.) mūrchchito harate vyādhīnmṛto jīvayati svayam | baddhaḥ khecharatāṃ dhatte raso vāyuścha pārvati

*O Pârvati! Mercury and breathing, when made steady,
destroy diseases and the dead himself comes to life (by
their means). By their (proper) control, moving in the
air is attained.*

28.) manaḥ sthairyaṃ sthiro vāyustato binduḥ sthiro bhavet | bindu-sthairyātsadā sattvaṃ piṇḍa-sthairyaṃ prajāyate

*The breathing is calmed when the mind becomes steady
and calm; and hence the preservation of bindu. The
preservation of this latter makes the satwa established in
the body.*

29.) indriyāṇāṃ mano nātho manonāthastu mārutaḥ | mārutasya layo nāthaḥ sa layo nādamāśritaḥ

Mind is the master of the senses, and the breath is the

*master of the mind. The breath in its turn is subordinate
to the laya (absorption), and that laya depends on the
nâda.*

30.) so|ayamevāstu mokṣhākhyo māstu vāpi matāntare | manaḥ-prāṇa-laye kaśchidānan-daḥ sampravartate

This very laya is what is called moksa, or, being a sectarian, you may not call it moksa; but when the mind becomes absorbed, a sort of ecstacy is experienced.

31.) pranaṣhṭa-śvāsa-niśvāsaḥ pradh-vasta-viṣhaya-ghrahaḥ | niścheṣhṭo nir-vikāraścha layo jayati yoghinām

*By the suspension of respiration and the annihilation of
the enjoyments of the senses, when the mind becomes
devoid of all the activities and remains changeless, then
the Yogî attains to the Laya Stage.*

32.) uchchinna-sarva-sangkalp-niḥśeṣhāśeṣha-cheṣhṭitaḥ | svāvaghamyo layaḥ ko|api jāyate vāgh-aghocharaḥ

*All the prominent desires being entirely finished, and
the body motionless, results in the absorption or laya,*

which is only known by the Self, and beyond the scope of words.

33.) yatra dṛṣhṭirlayastatra bhūtend-riya-sanātanī I sā śaktirjīva-bhūtānāṃ dve alakṣhye layaṃ ghate

Where the sight is directed, absorption occurs. That in which the elements, senses and shakti exist externally, which is in all living things, both ore dissolved in the characteristicless.

34.) layo laya iti prāhuḥ kīdṛśaṃ laya-lakṣhaṇam I apunar-vāsanotthānāllayo vishaya-vismṛtiḥ

Some say 'laya, laya' but what is the characteristic of laya or absorption? Laya is the non-recollection of the objects of the senses when the previous deep-rooted desires (and impressions) are non-recurrent.

35.) veda-śāstra-purāṇāni sāmānya-ghaṇikā iva I ekaiva śāmbhavī mudrā ghuptā ku-la-vadhūriva

The Vedas, shastras and Puranas are like common women, but shambhavi is secret like a woman of good heritage.

36.) atha śāmbhavī

antarlakṣhyam bahirdṛ̥ṣhṭirnimeṣhonme-

ṣha-varjitā | eṣhā sā śāmbhavī mudrā ve-

da-śāstreṣhu ghopitā

The Sâmbhavî Mudrâ.

*With internalized (one-pointed) awareness and external
gaze unblinking, that verily is shambhavi mudra, pre-
served in the Vedas.*

37.) antarlakṣhya-vilīna-chitta-pavano yoghī

yadā vartate dṛ̥ṣhṭyā niśchala-tārayā bahirad-

haḥ paśyannapaśyannapi | mudreyam khalu

śāmbhavī bhavati sā labdhā prasādādghuroḥ

śūnyāśūnya-vilakṣhaṇam sphurati tattattvam

padam śāmbhavam

*When the Yogî remains inwardly attentive to the Brah-
man, keeping the mind and the Prâna absorbed, and
the sight steady, as if seeing everything while in reality
seeing nothing outside, below, or above, verily then it is
called the Sâmbhavî Mudrâ, which is learnt by the fa-
vour of a guru. Whatever, wonderful, Sûnya or Asûnya
is perceived, is to be regarded as the manifestation of
that great Sambhû (Śiva.)*

**38.) śrī-śāmbhavyāścha khecharyā avast-
hā-dhāma-bhedataḥ I bhavechchitta-layā-
nandaḥ śūnye chit-sukha-rūpiṇi**

*The two states, the Sâmbhavî and the Khecharî, are
different because of their seats (being the heart and
the space between the eyebrows respectively); but both
cause happiness, for the mind becomes absorbed in the
Chita-sukha-Rupa-âtmana which is void.*

**39.) tāre jyotiṣhi saṃyojya kiṃchidunnamay-
edbhruvau I pūrva-yoghaṃ mano yuñjan-
nunmanī-kārakaḥ kṣhaṇāt**

*With perfect concentration, the pupils fixed on the light
by raising the eyebrows up a little, as from the previous-
ly described (shambhavi), mind is joined and instantly
unmani occurs.*

**40.) kechidāghama-jālena kechinnigha-
ma-sangkulaiḥ I kechittarkeṇa muhyanti
naiva jānanti tārakam**

*Some are devoted to the Vedas, some to Nigama, while
others are enwrapt in Logic, but none knows the value
of this mudrâ, which enables one to cross the ocean of
existence.*

41.) ardhonmīlita-lochanaḥ sthira-manā nāsāghra-dattekṣhaṇaś chandrārkāvapi līnatāmupanayannispanda-bhāvena yaḥ I jyotī-rūpamaśeṣha-bījamakhilaṃ dedīpyamānaṃ paraṃ tattvaṃ tat-padameti vastu paramaṃ vāchyaṃ kimatrādhikam

With steady calm mind and half closed eyes, fixed on the tip of the nose, stopping the Idâ and the Pingalâ without blinking, he who can see the light which is the all, the seed, the entire brilliant, great Tatwama, approaches Him, who is the great object. What is the use of more talk?

42.) divā na pūjayellinggham rātrau chaiva na pūjayet I sarvadā pūjayellinggham divārātri-nirodhataḥ

One should not meditate on the Linga (i.e., Âtman) in the day (i.e., while Sûrya or Pingalâ is working) or at night (when Idâ is working), but should always contemplate after restraining both.

43.) atha khecharī savya-dakṣhiṇa-nāḍī-stho madhye charati mārutaḥ I tiṣhṭhate khecharī mudrā tasminsthāne na saṃśayaḥ

The Khecharî.

When the prana which is in the right and left nadis mo-
ves m the middle nadi (sushumna) that is the condition
for khechari mudra.

44.) iḍā-pingghalayormadhye śūnyaṃ chaivā-
nilaṃ ghraset ǀ tiṣhṭhate khecharī mudrā
tatra satyaṃ punaḥ punaḥ

The fire (of shakti) being swallowed (suppressed) mid-
way between, ida and pingala, in that shoonya (of sus-
humna), is in truth the condition for khechari mudra.

45.) sūrchyāchandramasormadhye nirālam-
bāntare punaḥ ǀ saṃsthitā vyoma-chakre yā
sā mudrā nāma khecharī

That Mudrâ is called Khecharî which is performed in
the supportless space between the Sûrya and the Ch-
andra (the Idâ and the Pingalâ) and called the Vyoma
Chakra.

46.) somādyatroditā dhārā sākṣhātsā śiva-val-
labhā ǀ pūrayedatulāṃ divyāṃ suṣhumṇāṃ
paśchime mukhe

The Khecharî which causes the stream to flow from the Chandra (Śoma) is beloved of Śiva. The incomparable divine Susumnâ should be closed by the tongue drawn back.

47.) purastāchchaiva pūryeta niśchitā khecharī bhavet | abhyastā khecharī mudrāpyunmanī samprajāyate

It can be closed from the front also (by stopping the movements of the Prâna), and then surely it becomes the Khecharî. By practice, this Khecharî leads to Unmanî.

48.) bhruvormadhye śiva-sthānaṃ manastatra vilīyate | jñātavyaṃ tat-padaṃ turyaṃ tatra kālo na vidyate

In the middle of the Eyebrows is the place of Shiva, there the mind is quiescent. That state is known as turiya or the fourth dimension. There, time is unknown.

49.) abhyasetkhecharīṃ tāvadyāvatsyādyogha-nidritaḥ | samprāpta-yogha-nidrasya kālo nāsti kadāchana

The Khecharî should be practised till there is Yoga-nidrâ (Samâdhi). One who has induced Yoga-nidrâ, cannot fall a victim to death.

**50.) nirālambaṃ manaḥ kṛtvā na kiṃchida-
pi chintayet | sa-bāhyābhyantaraṃ vyomni
ghaṭavattiṣhṭhati dhruvam**

*Freeing the mind from all thoughts and thinking of
nothing, one should sit firmly like a pot in the space
(surrounded and filled with the ether).*

**51.) bāhya-vāyuryathā līnastathā madhyo na
saṃśayaḥ | sva-sthāne sthiratāmeti pavano
manasā saha**

*As the air, in and out of the body, remains unmoved, so
the breath with mind becomes steady in its place (i.e., in
Brahma randhra).*

**52.) evamabhyasyatastasya vāyu-mārghe
divāniśam | abhyāsājjīryate vāyurmanasta-
traiva līyate**

*By thus practising, night and day, the breathing is
brought under control, and, as the practice increases, the
mind becomes calm and steady.*

**53.) amṛtaiḥ plāvayeddehamāpāda-tala-mas-
takam | siddhyatyeva mahā-kāyo mahā-ba-
la-parākramaḥ**

By rubbing the body over with Amrita (exuding from the moon), from head to foot, one gets Mahâkâyâ, i.e., great strength and energy.

End of the Khecharî.

54.) śakti-madhye manaḥ kṛtvā śaktiṃ mā-nasa-madhyaghām | manasā mana ālokya dhārayetparamaṃ padam

Placing the mind into the Kundalini, and getting the latter into the mind, by looking upon the Buddhi (intellect) with mind (reflexively), the Param Pada (Brahma) should be obtained.

55.) kha-madhye kuru chātmānamātma-mad-hye cha khaṃ kuru | sarvaṃ cha kha-mayaṃ kṛtvā na kiṃchidapi chintayet

Keep the âtmâ inside the Kha (Brahma) and place Brahma inside your âtmâ. Having made everything pervaded with Kha (Brahma), think of nothing else.

56.) antaḥ śūnyo bahiḥ śūnyaḥ śūnyaḥ kum-bha ivāmbare | antaḥ pūrṇo bahiḥ pūrṇaḥ pūrṇaḥ kumbha ivārṇave

*One should become void in and void out, and voice like
a pot in the space. Full in and full outside, like a jar in
the ocean.*

57.) bāhya-chintā na kartavyā tathaivānta-ra-chintanam | sarva-chintāṃ parityajya na kiṃchidapi chintayet

*He should be neither of his inside nor of outside world;
and, leaving all thoughts, he should think of nothing.*

58.) sangkalpa-mātra-kalanaiva jaghatsam-aghraṃ sangkalpa-mātra-kalanaiva ma-no-vilāsaḥ | sangkalpa-mātra-matimutsṛja nirvikalpam āśritya niśchayamavāpnuhi rāma śāntim

*The whole of this world and all the schemes of the
mind are but the creations of thought. Discarding these
thoughts and taking leave of all conjectures, O Râma!
obtain peace.*

59.) karpūramanale yadvatsaindhavaṃ salile yathā | tathā sandhīyamānaṃ cha manas-tattve vilīyate

*As camphor disappears in fire, and rock salt in water, so
the mind united with the âtmâ loses its identity.*

**60.) jñeyaṃ sarvaṃ pratītaṃ cha jñānaṃ
cha mana uchyate | jñānaṃ jñeyaṃ samaṃ
naṣhṭaṃ nānyaḥ panthā dvitīyakaḥ**

*When the knowable, and the knowledge, are both
destroyed equally, then there is no second way (i.e.,
Duality is destroyed).*

**61.) mano-dṝśyamidaṃ sarvaṃ yat-
kiṃchitsa-charācharam | manaso hyun-
manī-bhāvāddvaitaṃ naivolabhyate**

*All this movable and immovable world is mind. When
the mind has attained to the unmanî avasthâ, there
is no dwaita (from the absence of the working of the
mind.)*

**62.) jñeya-vastu-parityāghādvilayaṃ yāti
mānasam | manaso vilaye jāte kaivalyama-
vaśiṣhyate**

*Mind disappears by removing the knowable, and, on its
disappearance, âtmâ only remains behind.*

**63.) evaṃ nānā-vidhopāyāḥ samy-
aksvānubhavānvitāḥ | samādhi-mārghāḥ
kathitāḥ pūrvāchāryairmahātmabhiḥ**

The high-souled Âchâryas (Teachers) of yore gained ex-perience in the various methods of Samâdhi themselves, and then they preached them to others.

64.) suṣhumṇāyai kuṇḍalinyai sudhāyai ch-andra-janmane I manonmanyai namastubhy-am mahā-śaktyai chid-ātmane

Salutations to Thee, O Susumnâ, to Thee O Kundalinî, to Thee O Sudhâ, born of Chandra, to Thee O Manom-nanî! to Thee O great power, energy and the intelligent spirit.

65.) aśakya-tattva-bodhānāṃ mūḍhānāmapi sammatam I proktaṃ ghorakṣha-nāthena nādopāsanamuchyate

I will describe now the practice of anâhata nâda, as pro-pounded by Goraksa Nâtha, for the benefit of those who are unable to understand the principles of knowledge—a method, which is liked by the ignorant also.

66.) śrī-ādināthena sa-pāda-koṭi-laya-prakārāḥ kathitā jayanti I nādānusandhānakamekame-va manyāmahe mukhyatamaṃ layānām

Âdinâtha propounded 1¼ crore methods of trance, and

they are all extant. Of these, the hearing of the anâhata
nâda is the Only one, the chief, in my opinion.

67.) muktāsane sthito yoghī mudrāṃ sand-
hāya śāmbhavīm | śṛṇuyāddakṣhiṇe karṇe
nādamantāsthamekadhīḥ

Sitting with Mukta Âsana and with the Sâmbhavî Ma-
dill, the Yogî should hear the sound inside his right ear,
with collected mind.

68.) śravaṇa-puṭa-nayana-yughala
ghrāṇa-mukhānāṃ nirodhanaṃ kāryam |
śuddha-suṣhumṇā-saraṇau sphuṭamamalaḥ
śrūyate nādaḥ

The ears, the eyes, the nose, and the mouth should be
closed and then the clear sound is heard in the passa-
ge of the Susumnâ which has been cleansed of all its
impurities.

69.) ārambhaścha ghaṭaśchaiva tathā pa-
richayo|api cha | niṣhpattiḥ sarva-yogheṣhu
syādavasthā-chatuṣhṭayam

In all the Yogas, there are four states: (1) ârambha or the
preliminary, (2) Ghata, or the state of a jar, (3) Pa-
richaya (known), (4) nispatti (consumate.)

70.) atha ārambhāvasthā
brahma-ghrantherbhavedbhedo hyānandaḥ
śūnya-sambhavaḥ | vichitraḥ kvaṇako de-
he|anāhataḥ śrūyate dhvaniḥ

Ârambha Avasthâ.

When the Brahma granthi (in the heart) is pierced through by Prânâyâma, then a sort of happiness is experienced in the vacuum of the heart, and the anâhat sounds, like various tinkling sounds of ornaments, are heard in the body.

71.) divya-dehaścha tejasvī divya-ghandhas-
tvaroghavān | sampūrṇa-hṛdayaḥ śūnya
ārambhe yoghavānbhavet

In the ârambha, a Yogî's body becomes divine, glowing, healthy, and emits a divine swell. The whole of his heart becomes void.

72.) atha ghaṭāvasthā
dvitīyāyāṃ ghaṭīkṛtya vāyurbhavati mad-
hyaghaḥ | dṛḍhāsano bhavedyoghī jñānī
deva-samastadā

The Ghata Avasthâ.

In the second stage, the airs are united into one and begin moving in the middle channel. The Yogî's posture becomes firm, and he becomes wise like a god.

73.) viṣhṇu-ghranthestato bhedātparamā-nanda-sūchakaḥ | atiśūnye vimardaścha bherī-śabdastadā bhavet

By this means the Vishu knot (in the throat) is pierced which is indicated by highest pleasure experienced, And then the Bherî sound (like the beating of a kettle drain) is evolved in the vacuum in the throat.

74.) atha parichayāvasthā tṛtīyāyāṃ tu vijñeyo vihāyo mardala-dhva-niḥ | mahā-śūnyaṃ tadā yāti sarva-sidd-hi-samāśrayam

The Parichaya Avasthâ.

In the third stage, the sound of a drum is known to arise in tie Sûnya between the eyebrows, and then the Vâyu goes to the Mahâśûnya, which is the home of all the siddhîs.

**75.) chittānandaṃ tadā jitvā sahajānan-
da-sambhavaḥ | doṣha-duḥkha-jarā-vyād-
hi-kṣhudhā-nidrā-vivarjitaḥ**

*Conquering, then, the pleasures of the mind, ecstacy is
spontaneously produced which is devoid of evils, pains,
old age, disease, hunger and sleep.*

**76.) atha niṣhpatty-avasthā
rudra-ghranthiṃ yadā bhittvā śar-
va-pīṭha-ghato|anilaḥ | niṣhpattau vaiṇavaḥ
śabdaḥ kvaṇad-vīṇā-kvaṇo bhavet**

The Nishpatty Avasthâ.

*When the Rudra granthi is pierced and the air enters the
seat of the Lord (the space between the eyebrows), then
the perfect sound like that of a flute is produced.*

**77.) ekībhūtaṃ tadā chittaṃ rāja-yoghābhid-
hānakam | sṛṣhṭi-saṃhāra-kartāsau yog-
hīśvara-samo bhavet**

*The union of the mind and the sound is called the
Râja-Yoga. The (real) Yogî becomes the creator and
destroyer of the universe, like God.*

**78.) astu vā māstu vā muktiratraivākhaṇḍi-
taṃ sukham I layodbhavamidaṃ saukhyaṃ
rāja-yoghādavāpyate**

*Perpetual Happiness is achieved by this; I do not care
if the mukti be not attained. This happiness, resulting
from absorption [in Brahma], is obtained by means of
Raja-Yoga.*

**79.) rāja-yoghamajānantaḥ kevalaṃ
haṭha-karmiṇaḥ I etānabhyāsino manye
prayāsa-phala-varjitān**

*Those who are ignorant of the Râja-Yoga and practise
only the Hatha-Yoga, will, in my opinion, waste their
energy fruitlessly.*

**80.) unmany-avāptaye śīghraṃ bhrū-dhyā-
naṃ mama saṃmatam I rāja-yogha-padaṃ
prāptuṃ sukhopāyo|alpa-chetasām I sadyaḥ
pratyaya-sandhāyī jāyate nādajo layaḥ**

*Contemplation on the space between the eyebrows is,
in my opinion, best for accomplishing soon the Unmanî
state. For people of small intellect, it is a very easy
method for obtaining perfection in the Raja-Yoga. The
Laya produced by nâda, at once gives experience (of
spiritual powers).*

**81.) nādānusandhāna-samādhi-bhājāṃ yog-
hīśvarāṇāṃ hṛdi vardhamānam | ānandame-
kaṃ vachasāmaghamyaṃ jānāti taṃ śrī-ghu-
runātha ekaḥ**

*The happiness which increases in the hearts of Yogiśwa-
ras, who have gained success in Samâdhi by means of
attention to the nâda, is beyond description, and is
known to Śri Gurû Nâtha alone.*

**82.) karṇau pidhāya hastābhyāṃ yaḥ śṛṇoti
dhvaniṃ muniḥ | tatra chittaṃ sthirīkuryā-
dyāvatsthira-padaṃ vrajet**

*The sound which a muni hears by closing his ears with
his fingers, should be heard attentively, till the mind
becomes steady in it.*

**83.) abhyasyamāno nādo|ayaṃ bāhyamāvṛṇu-
te dhvanim | pakṣhādvikṣhepamakhilaṃ
jitvā yoghī sukhī bhavet**

*By practising with this nâda, all other external sounds
are stopped. The Yogî becomes happy by overcoming all
distractions within 15 days.*

**84.) śrūyate prathamābhyāse nādo nānā-vid-
ho mahān | tato|abhyāse vardhamāne śrūya-
te sūkṣhma-sūkṣhmakaḥ**

*In the beginning, the sounds heard are of great variety
and very loud; but, as the practice increases, they beco-
me more and more subtle.*

**85.) ādau jaladhi-jīmūta-bherī-jharjhara-sam-
bhavāḥ ' | madhye mardala-śangkhotthā
ghaṇṭā-kāhalajāstathā**

*In the first stage, the sounds are surging, thundering like
the beating of kettle drums and jingling ones. In the in-
termediate stage, they are like those produced by conch,
Mridanga, bells, &c.*

**86.) ante tu kingkiṇī-vaṃśa-vīṇā-bhramara-
niḥsvanāḥ | iti nānāvidhā nādāḥ śrūyante
deha-madhyaghāḥ**

*In the last stage, the sounds resemble those from tinklets,
flute, bee, &c. These various kinds of sounds are heard
as being produced in the body.*

**87.) mahati śrūyamāṇe|api megha-bhery-ādi-
ke dhvanau | tatra sūkṣhmātsūkṣhmataraṃ
nādameva parāmṛśet**

Though hearing loud sounds like those of thunder, kettle drums, etc. one should practise with the subtle sounds also.

88.) ghanamutsṝjya vā sūkṣhme sūkṣhmam-utsṝjya vā ghane | ramamāṇamapi kṣhiptaṃ mano nānyatra chālayet

Leaving the loudest, taking up the subtle one, and leaving the subtle one, taking up the loudest, thus practising, the distracted mind does not wander elsewhere.

89.) yatra kutrāpi vā nāde laghati prathamaṃ manaḥ | tatraiva susthirībhūya tena sārdhaṃ vilīyate

Wherever the mind attaches itself first, it becomes steady there; and then it becomes absorbed in it.

90.) makarandaṃ pibanbhṝngghī ghandhaṃ nāpekṣhate yathā | nādāsaktaṃ tathā chit-taṃ viṣhayānnahi kāngkṣhate

Just as a bee, drinking sweet juice, does not care for the smell of the flower; so the mind, absorbed in the nâda, does not desire the objects of enjoyment.

**91.) mano-matta-ghajendrasya vishayodyā-
na-chāriṇaḥ | samartho|ayaṃ niyamane
nināda-niśitāngkuśaḥ**

*The mind, like an elephant habituated to wander in the
garden of enjoyments, is capable of being controlled by
the sharp goad of anâhata nâda.*

**92.) baddhaṃ tu nāda-bandhena manaḥ san-
tyakta-chāpalam | prayāti sutarāṃ sthairyaṃ
chinna-pakṣhaḥ khagho yathā**

*The mind, captivated in the snare of nâda, gives up all
its activity; and, like a bird with clipped wings, becomes
calm at once.*

**93.) sarva-chintāṃ parityajya sāvadhānena
chetasā | nāda evānusandheyo yogha-sām-
rājyamichchhatā**

*Those desirous of the kingdom of Yoga, should take up
the practice of hearing the anâhata nâda, with mind
collected and free from all cares.*

**94.) nādo|antaranggha-saranggha-bandhane
vāghurāyate | antaranggha-kurangghasya
vadhe vyādhāyate|api cha**

Nada is the snare for catching the mind; and, when it is caught like a deer, it can be killed also like it.

95.) antarangghasya yamino vājinaḥ parig-hāyate | nādopāsti-rato nityamavadhāryā hi yoghinā

Nâda is the bolt of the stable door for the horse (the minds of the Yogîs). A Yogî should determine to practise constantly in the hearing of the nâda sounds.

96.) baddhaṃ vimukta-chāñchalyaṃ nā-da-ghandhaka-jāraṇāt | manaḥ-pāradamāp-noti nirālambākhya-kheḷaṭanam

Mind gets the properties of calcined mercury. When deprived of its unsteadiness it is calcined, combined with the sulphur of nâda, and then it roams like it in tine supportless âkâśa or Brahma. 95.

97.) nāda-śravaṇataḥ kṣhipramantarangg-ha-bhujangghamam | vismṛtaya sarva-mekāghraḥ kutrachinnahi dhāvati

The mind is like a serpent, forgetting all its unsteadiness by hearing the nâda, it does not run away anywhere.

**98.) kāṣhṭhe pravartito vahniḥ kāṣhṭhena
saha śāmyati | nāde pravartitaṃ chittaṃ
nādena saha līyate**

*The fire, catching firewood, is extinguished along with
it (after burning it up); and so the mind also, working
with the nâda, becomes latent along with it.*

**99.) ghaṇṭādināda-sakta-stabdhāntaḥ-ka-
raṇa-hariṇasya | praharaṇamapi sukaraṃ
syāchchara-sandhāna-pravīṇaśchet**

*The antahkarana (mind), like a deer, becomes absorbed
and motionless on hearing the sound of hells, etc. and
then it is very easy for an expert archer to kill it.*

**100.) anāhatasya śabdasya dhvanirya upa-
labhyate | dhvanerantarghataṃ jñeyaṃ jñey-
asyāntarghataṃ manaḥ | manastatra layaṃ
yāti tadviṣhṇoḥ paramaṃ padam**

*The knowable interpenetrates the anâhata sound which
is heard, and the mind interpenetrates the knowable.
The mind becomes absorbed there, which is the seat of
the all-pervading, almighty Lord.*

101.) tāvadākāśa-sangkalpo yāvachchabdaḥ pravartate I niḥśabdaṃ tat-paraṃ brahma paramāteti ghīyate

So long as the sounds continue, there is the idea of âkâśa. When they disappear, then it is called Para Brahma, Paramâtmana.

102.) yatkiṃchinnāda-rūpeṇa śrūyate śaktireva sā I yastattvānto nirākāraḥ sa eva parameśvaraḥ

Whatever is heard in the form of nâda, is the śakti (power). That which is formless, the final state of the Tatwas, is tile Parameśwara.

103.) iti nādānusandhānam sarve haṭha-layopāyā rājayoghasya siddhaye I rāja-yogha-samārūḍhaḥ puruṣhaḥ kāla-vañchakaḥ

All the methods of Hatha are meant for gaining success in the Raja-Yoga; for, the man, who is well-established in the Raja-Yoga, overcomes death.

104.) tattvaṃ bījaṃ haṭhaḥ kshetramaudāsīnyaṃ jalaṃ tribhiḥ I unmanī kalpa-latikā sadya eva pravartate

Tatwa is the seed, Hatha the field; and Indifference (Vairâgya) the water. By the action of these three, the creeper Unmanî thrives very rapidly.

105.) sadā nādānusandhānātkṣhīyante pā-pa-saṃchayāḥ | nirañjane vilīyete niśchitaṃ chitta-mārutau

All the accumulations of sins are destroyed by practising always with the nâda; and the mind and the airs do certainly become latent in the colorless (Paramâtmana).

106.) śangkha-dundhubhi-nādaṃ cha na śṛṇoti kadāchana | kāṣhṭhavajjāyate deha unmanyāvasthayā dhruvam

Such a one. does not hear the noise of the conch and Dundubhi. Being in the Unmanî avasthâ, his body becomes like a piece of wood.

107.) sarvāvasthā-vinirmuktaḥ sarva-chintā-vivarjitaḥ | mṛtavattiṣhṭhate yoghī sa mukto nātra saṃśayaḥ

There is no doubt, such a Yogî becomes free from all states, from all cares, and remains like one dead.

**108.) khādyate na cha kālena bādhyate na
cha karmaṇā | sādhyate na sa kenāpi yoghī
yuktaḥ samādhinā**

*He is not devoured by death, is not bound by his
actions. The Yogî who is engaged in Samâdhi is over-
powered by none.*

**109.) na ghandhaṃ na rasaṃ rūpaṃ na cha
sparśaṃ na niḥsvanam | nātmānaṃ na pa-
raṃ vetti yoghī yuktaḥ samādhinā**

*The Yogî, engaged in Samâdhi, feels neither smell, taste,
color, touch, sound, nor is conscious of his own self.*

**110.) chittaṃ na suptaṃ nojāghratsmṛ-
ti-vismṛti-varjitam | na chāstameti nodeti
yasyāsau mukta eva saḥ**

*He whose mind is neither sleeping, waking, remembe-
ring, destitute of memory, disappearing nor appearing,
is liberated.*

**111.) na vijānāti śītoṣhṇaṃ na duḥkhaṃ na
sukhaṃ tathā | na mānaṃ nopamānaṃ cha
yoghī yuktaḥ samādhinā**

*He feels neither heat, cold, pain, pleasure, respect nor
disrespect. Such a Yogî is absorbed in Samâdhi.*

112.) svastho jāghradavasthāyāṃ suptava-dyo|avatiṣhṭhate | niḥśvāsochchvāsa-hī-naścha niśchitaṃ mukta eva saḥ

*He who, though awake, appears like one sleeping, and is
without inspiration and expiration, is certainly free.*

113.) avadhyaḥ sarva-śastrāṇāmaśakyaḥ sar-va-dehinām | aghrāhyo mantra-yantrāṇāṃ yoghī yuktaḥ samādhinā

*The Yogî, engaged in Samâdhi, cannot be killed by any
instrument, and is beyond the controlling power of bein-
gs. He is beyond the reach of incantations and charms.*

114.) yāvadvidurna bhavati dṛḍhaḥ prāṇa-vā-ta-prabandhāt | yāvaddhyāne saha-ja-sadṛśaṃ jāyate naiva tattvaṃ tāvajjñānaṃ vadati tadidaṃ dambha-mithyā-pralāpaḥ

*As long as the Prâna does not enter and flow in the
middle channel and the vindu does not become firm by
the control of the movements of the Prâna; as long as the
mind does not assume the form of Brahma without any*

effort in contemplation, so long all the talk of knowledge and wisdom is merely the nonsensical babbling of a mad man.

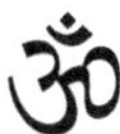

iti haṭha-yogha-pradīpikāyāṃ samād-
hi-lakṣhaṇaṃ nāma chaturthopadeśaḥ |

THE END.